GEMSTONE REFLEXOLOGY

Nora Kircher

Translated from the German by
Nikolas Win Myint

Healing Arts Press
Rochester, Vermont

Healing Arts Press
One Park Street
Rochester, Vermont 05767
www.HealingArtsPress.com

Healing Arts Press is a division of Inner Traditions International

Originally published in German under the title *Edelstein-Akupressur: Schmerzfrei und gesünder mit dem Kristall-Stab* by Neue Erde Verlag GmbH, Saarbrücken, Germany
First U.S. edition published in 2006 by Healing Arts Press

Note to the reader: This book is intended as an informational guide. The remedies, approaches, and techniques described herein are meant to supplement, and not to be a substitute for, professional medical care or treatment. They should not be used to treat a serious ailment without prior consultation with a qualified health care professional.

LIBRARY OF CONGRESS CATALOGING-IN-PUBLICATION DATA
Kircher, Nora, 1956–
    [Edelstein-Akupressur. English]
    Gemstone reflexology / Nora Kircher ; translated from the German by Nikolas Win Myint.
        p. cm.
    "Originally published in German under the title: Edelstein-Akupressur: Schmerzfrei und gesünder mit dem Kristall-Stab by Neue Erde Verlag GmbH, Saarbrücken, Germany."
    Summary: "An innovative and holistic approach that combines the healing powers of gemstones with reflexology and acupressure"—Provided by publisher.
    Includes index.
    ISBN-13: 978-1-59477-121-7 (pbk.)
    ISBN-10: 1-59477-121-9 (pbk.)
    1. Gemstones—Therapeutic use. 2. Reflexology (Therapy) 3. Acupressure. I. Title.
    RZ560.K5313 2006
    615.8'224—dc22
                                                                        2006011027

Printed and bound in China by Regent

10   9   8   7   6   5   4   3   2   1

Photos by Christopher Cornwell

Text design by Jonathan Desautels
Text layout by Virginia Scott Bowman
This book was typeset in Sabon and Gil Sans with Warnock Pro as the display typeface

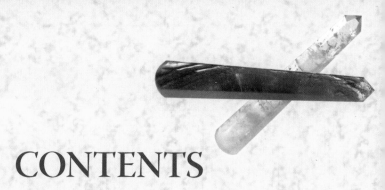

CONTENTS

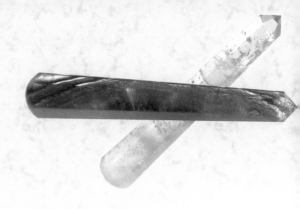

INTRODUCTION

The entire human body is reflected on some of its parts, including the ears, feet, and back. Those familiar with these reflections of the body on individual body parts can utilize this knowledge to successfully treat pain and many other health conditions.

In my own practice in Germany, I combine the healing energies of gemstones with the well-established therapeutic principles of reflexology and acupressure. These therapies, traditionally administered with the hands or acupuncture needles, are wonderfully suited for gemstone massage techniques.

People come to my practice with a wide range of ailments, and I can help almost all of them with gemstone reflexology and acupressure. All of my acupuncture textbooks remain largely unread on the shelf, because I use a diagram that depicts the human body reflected upside down on the ear, in the embryo position. Using this diagram, one can quickly learn where specific body parts are located on the ear.

The gem stick treatment methods I discuss in this book allow you to direct the specific healing power of eight different gemstones to activate designated acupressure points and reflexology zones on the body. My approach is holistic, with a goal of triggering the body's own self-healing energies. Holistic treatment aims to treat not just a specific symptom or ailment, but the whole person. When used for whole body treatment, gem stick acupressure and reflexology can be a valuable part of holistic treatment for any ailment. While my focus in this book is on how to use gem sticks, I have included a few additional suggestions for supportive therapies in each of my treatment protocols, including simple homeopathic and herbal remedies and other natural treatments.

In my work as an instructor, I am always happy to observe how quickly my students become successful with my techniques. You will see that once you understand the basic principles of acupressure and reflexology and have gained some practice with them, your gem sticks will bring you a great deal of joy and healing.

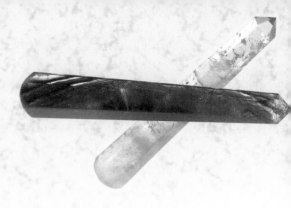

THE
GEM STICKS

Gem sticks, also known as crystal tips or gem tips, are an essential part of my healing practice. Used in combination with my reflexology and acupressure techniques, I have found gemstones to be invaluable aids for successfully treating a wide range of ailments, including pain of all kinds.

Gemstones bring a wonderful healing energy to reflexology and acupressure treatment. Each stone has different healing attributes, and some are better suited for certain purposes than others. However, as a basic principle, you can carry out any reflexology or acupressure treatment with any type of stone. In theory, you can also perform ear acupressure using a paper clip bent into an open position or a similarly sharp object, although you will not get the benefits of the strong, positive energy provided by gemstones. When you use the pointed end of a gem stick, you may find that gently touching the area to be treated is sufficient treatment. With other sharp objects, it may be necessary to stimulate the point for a much longer period of time, which may be painful for the recipient without providing the same beneficial effects.

Gem sticks bundle energy in the pointed end of the stone and distribute energy broadly through the blunt end. This energy has different intensity and varying effects depending on the type of stone you are using. Moreover, different gem sticks made from the same type of stone may also have slightly different effects. For this reason, I describe only approximate guidelines for the effects of each type of stone.

When you purchase a gem stick, make sure that the stone has both a blunt and a sharp (pointed) end. The sharp end should be neither broken nor rounded off. You may want to purchase one gem stick to begin with until you have become proficient in the treatment basics, at which point it can be exciting to experiment with the subtleties of the gems' different healing energies. For optimal success with your therapy, it is essential that the stone be authentic.

You will find more on the topic of authentic gemstones and the healing effects of different types of gems in books such as *Crystal Power, Crystal Healing* by Michael Gienger and *The Crystal Bible* by Judy Hall.

When you are not using your gem sticks, don't hide them in a drawer. Leave them out and enjoy their beauty.

Amethyst

This purple, semitransparent stone is perceived as spiritual and is valued for its beautiful, intense color. Amethyst emanates calm. Its soothing aura promotes sleep, calms the soul, and alleviates pain.

Because almost all illness entails pain and anxiety, the calming and pain-relieving attributes of amethyst make it one of the most important healing stones. In general, anxiety in the body can lead to tense muscles, which can cause back pain and headache. Amethyst can help alleviate this kind of pain as well as pain due to infection, such as severe bronchitis.

Amethyst is extremely beneficial for the mind and psyche, helping to calm, balance, and focus the thoughts and emotions. It is considered one of the most spiritual gemstones and is useful in helping people overcome addictions.

Aventurine

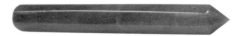

Aventurine is a popular stone especially liked by children. Its soft shine gives it an interesting structure. Green aventurine has a light- to medium-green color that is reminiscent of spring.

Green is the most important color in nature. When we take a walk in the green of nature or rest there, we gather strength, harmony, and a sense of relaxation. This is why green aventurine helps bring about a general sense of well-being.

Aventurine is especially effective for mental tension and for alleviating pain. It balances blood pressure and is a useful addition to any holistic treatment for cardiovascular problems. Aventurine is also useful for migraines, sinus problems, and skin eruptions.

Fluorite

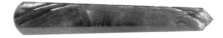

This multicolored, almost transparent gem is often used as a learning aid. You will see purple, green, and sometimes white structures connected alongside one another in this stone. Perhaps this is why fluorite enhances concentration and encourages interaction between the two halves of the brain. The right side of our brain controls our creative impulses and the left side abstract thinking, so it is important that the two sides work together.

Fluorite is an important stone for the treatment of infections and has a healing effect on the skin and mucous membranes. Mucous membranes line the mouth and all other hollow internal organs, such as the esophagus, stomach, intestines, and the breathing organs. For this reason, fluorite is beneficial against colds and flu and sinus infections. It is helpful against arthritis pain as well as nerve-related pain, such as shingles.

Heliotrope

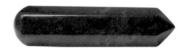

The saying "Opposites attract" is appropriate for heliotrope, and those who like strong colors will probably be attracted to this stone. The deep green stone, also known as bloodstone, contains striking, complementary red dots.

Heliotrope reminds some people of the green summertime, during which we can find red berries. Green helps fortify the body's defenses, while red gives strength, warmth, and fire. Blood contains iron, which is essential for life and is reflected in the red parts of this stone also containing iron.

Use heliotrope to regenerate and boost the body's immune system defenses, to treat menstrual problems, and to promote relaxation. Heliotrope helps detoxify the body and is also useful for conditions involving the blood and circulation.

Rock Crystal

Rock crystals, especially very clear ones, emanate a great deal of energy. Energy is stimulating for people who are weak due to illness and can be helpful for symptoms of paralysis.

Rock crystal (also known as clear quartz crystal) is one of the most powerful healing stones and is useful against nearly all illnesses. For this reason, it is a good gemstone to start with. It stimulates the immune system and helps balance body functions. Clear rock crystals generate clarity and cleanse both spirit and body. Cleansing is important for any illness, especially if caused by infection. Even the ancient Greeks attributed healing powers to rock crystal.

Rose Quartz

Women and girls and those attracted to softness often particularly like the transparent pink rose quartz. The color pink is composed of two colors: red (the color of blood) and white (a color associated with clarity). Blood contains important immune system components, such as white blood cells, that help cleanse the tissues of the body. Thus, it is important that sick tissue have good blood circulation.

Rose quartz is helpful for the heart and whole cardiovascular system and helps enhance good blood circulation. Rose quartz also can be used to treat menstrual problems, as well as chest and lung disorders. If the energy of rock crystal is too strong, rose quartz offers a good alternative.

On the emotional level, rose quartz helps heal heartache, grief, and sadness. It is considered one of the best healing stones for emotional pain of all kinds.

Rutile Quartz

Rutile quartz (sometimes called rutilated quartz) is rock crystal that contains titanium. Thus, the stone combines the strength of rock crystal with the purity and strength of titanium oxide.

Rutile quartz is easily differentiated from rock crystal: If you hold it against the light, you will see in the stone fine titanium needles ranging in color from dark yellow to copper red. Pure titanium is used in orthopedic medicine and in the eyeglass industry for its strength.

Rutile quartz releases tension, improves mood, and provides stability. This is a particularly helpful stone for depression and anxiety. In the stone, the needles are connected to form fine branches reminiscent of the bronchial tubes in our lungs, reflecting the fact that rutile quartz is useful for treating lung ailments.

Sodalite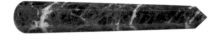

Sodalite is a dark blue, opaque stone sometimes crossed by white lines. Because this stone has a strong color and does not reveal its inside, it gives a sense of self-confidence. Self-confidence, in turn, can have calming effects, much as the blue color of this stone is calming and cooling.

The calming, cooling effects of this stone can help with insomnia, fever, and infection. Sodalite also helps boost immune system function and is useful against disorders of the throat and digestive tract.

Cleansing Your Stones

Wash your gem stick under running water after each use. If you used massage oil in your gem stick treatment, wash with a little bit of soap; otherwise, use plain water. You should also periodically do an energetic cleansing using salt or sunlight.

The easiest way to do an energetic cleansing is to place the stone in a bowl filled with salt and leave it there for a few hours. The salt can be used multiple times. You can also cleanse the stone by placing it on a sunny windowsill and allowing it to sit there for a few hours. Do not leave the stone in the sunlight for longer than a few hours. If you know how to use a pendulum or hand rod, you can verify the success of your cleansing with one of these tools. There is more information on using hand rods and pendulums with gemstone reflexology in the following chapter in the Choosing the Right Stone and Finding the Right Spot to Treat sections.

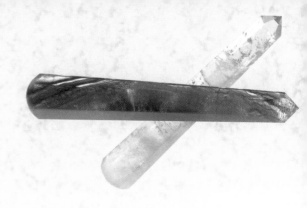

TYPES OF THERAPY

In my healing practice, I use gem sticks to enhance my ear acupressure, foot reflexology, body reflexology, and reflexology massage techniques. Through the years, I have had great success using these techniques to treat everything from musculoskeletal pain to illnesses affecting the internal organs. I frequently use acupressure and reflexology techniques in combination. For example, I have excellent results treating back pain with a combination of ear acupressure, body acupressure, and reflexology massage.

It is essential to consult a doctor to get a proper diagnosis for any ailment with an unknown cause, particularly for symptoms or illnesses that have persisted for an extended period of time. But whatever the diagnosis, you can support the healing process and relieve pain using gem stick acupressure and reflexology techniques. The therapies I describe in this book not only alleviate pain and other symptoms, but also encourage the body to deal with the cause of illness through its own healing powers. As a simple example, acupressure can stimulate blood circulation in an ailing body part and thus help the body eliminate toxins or bacteria in the injured tissue.

As with any healing practice, although it may be tempting to try to help people outside of your family, this may be risky if you are not a trained health care practitioner.

Treatment Basics

While treatment with a gem stick is not always enough to effect a cure in itself, such treatment will always support the body's healing process. Gemstones cannot heal all illnesses, especially severe or life-threatening diseases, but can in most cases help alleviate any accompanying pain.

When used to treat an injury—for example, a bruise, sprain, or even a broken bone—gem stick acupressure relieves pain and supports the healing process. I have had patients in my practice with such severe back pain that doctors suspected a slipped disk. In most cases, the pain was so much better after one ear acupressure treatment that further examinations became unnecessary. In most cases, a few acupressure treatments sufficed to prompt a full recovery.

For acute illnesses, daily treatments—sometimes, several treatments a day—can effectively speed healing. For chronic ailments, regular acupressure twice a week over an extended period of time can alleviate symptoms and heal illness. Exactly how often and for how long you apply these treatments will be determined by the progress you see.

When you see directions such as "treat for 20 to 30 seconds" in treatment instructions, it is not necessary to consult a stopwatch. Count it out—you don't have to be precise to the last second.

Ideally, the recipient will be comfortably seated or lying down for acupressure treatment. However, I have had success in situations in which sitting or lying down was not possible: for example, in the case of nausea after a plane landing. I once successfully treated a friend's nausea with ear acupressure while we were standing around waiting for our bags.

For reflexology treatment of points on the body, feet, and back, the recipient should be lying down. Compared with ear acupressure, one drawback to these therapies is that some clothing or at least the shoes must be removed. Especially for older people, this can be a difficult and time-consuming undertaking. In contrast, the ears, hands, and face are easily accessible.

Self-treatment with Gem Sticks

With a little agility and practice, you may find that you are able to perform acupressure and reflexology to treat your own pain and illness. Ear acupressure is especially well suited for self-treatment, and points around the thumb and on the face are also easily reached. Foot reflexology may be more difficult to perform on yourself, since it can be hard to reach the soles of the feet.

Experience has shown that better results are usually achieved when reflexology and acupressure are administered by another person. Each person reacts differently, however, so it is worth experimenting for yourself. In some cases, self-treatment may actually yield better results, because you can easily locate and keep the stone on the precise spot that is hurting.

Working with Pain

Pain accompanies most illnesses, and for good reason. Pain warns us about injury and alerts us to the presence of infection. When we touch something hot with our fingers, pain prevents us from getting burned more badly. Without conscious thought, our reflexes kick in and we let go of the hot object. Pain ensures that we rest ourselves and take action against its cause.

Pain is a component of most infections. Even a small infection in a single joint can be extremely painful. If this were not the case, we might continue to strain the joint until it is destroyed and thus unusable.

Health conditions that do not cause immediate pain—for example, high blood sugar and elevated cholesterol levels—show us the consequences of a missing warning from the body. Such problems are often discovered only after they have caused further damage.

Almost every infection is accompanied by the same symptoms of inflammation: pain, redness, swelling, heat, and impaired function. In medical terms, the names for such illnesses usually end with the suffix -*itis*. Familiar examples include bronchitis (inflammation of the mucous membranes of the bronchial tubes), sinusitis (inflammation of the sinuses), tonsillitis (inflammation of the tonsils), and arthritis (inflammation of the joints).

For many (but not all) ailments, the cause may not be located in the same place in which the pain surfaces. If you do not treat the cause, the patient will not become truly well. Tension headaches provide a simple example. A pain reliever may help with the pain, but it will not address the cause of the problem. As long as the cause is not addressed, the symptom—in this case the headache—will recur. Tensions, in turn, have their own causes, which require treatment in their own right.

Using Pain to Guide Therapy

There are points on the ears, feet, back, hands, and face that correspond to specific parts of the body. When the points on the ears and feet are in need of treatment, they are sensitive to pain and have a different feel to them. Body acupressure points do not reflect pain in this way; they correspond in a different and more complicated way to the painful or ill areas of the body. To locate these points, you will have to rely entirely on the diagrams provided. The key to success with acupressure and reflexology lies in locating the right points and treating them for an appropriate length of time. Note that this can be uncomfortable for the person you are treating, so always be gentle with your gem stick.

Before beginning treatment, ask the recipient to consciously feel his or her pain—for example, to focus on the intensity of the pain felt in a joint. Pay attention to flexibility and range of motion, both of which are often reduced as a result of pain or illness. Your partner's perception of his or her symptoms is an important tool that will guide you in ascertaining the success of your treatment.

During treatment, check in frequently with your partner to ask how he or she is feeling—whether or not the pain has subsided or changed in any way. You may have to ask your partner to move the ailing body part or to get up and walk around for this. Checking with your partner about his or her pain will also help you determine how long to treat each point.

During acupressure, the painful or ill body part will often feel warm or tingling. These are both good signs that the therapy is working. Sometimes acupressure can lead to an initial worsening of symptoms. Luckily this happens only rarely, but when it does happen, don't be discouraged. Wait a few minutes and the pain will subside. If, as the pain decreases, your partner notes that the painful part feels better than before treatment, treat the same point again.

Ear Acupressure

The body is reflected upside down in the ear. If you divide the ear into a lower and an upper half, you can—with just a few exceptions—assume that the lower half of the ear corresponds to the upper half of the body and the upper half of the ear to the lower half of the body.

The head is reflected in the earlobe, which is why all problems affecting the head (including headaches, sinus infections, and toothaches) are treated there. In the middle and upper part of the auricle (the external ear structure) are all of the internal organs. The arms and legs are distributed across the rest of the upper auricle. Familiarize yourself with the location of different parts of the body as depicted in the diagram shown here. With a little practice, you will soon know even without the diagram where to find the areas you want to treat.

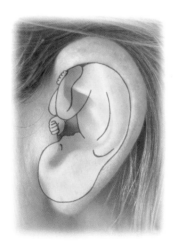

Diagram of an embryo of about two months old, reflected upside down on the ear. Although the body is not precisely aligned with the ear, this visualization can help you more easily understand and thus remember the general topography for ear acupressure.

The developing fetus is called an embryo during the first two months after conception. At this stage, the head is disproportionately large and the extremities (limbs) are small. The organs of the body are formed during this stage of growth.

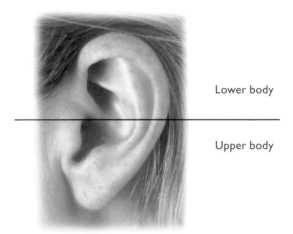

Lower body

Upper body

Application

For most people, pains in the right half of the body have to be treated in the right ear. Only rarely will you find the points to be treated on the opposite side, in the other ear. I always perform ear acupressure on both sides of the body, but longer and more carefully on the ear on the side of the body on which the problem is located. Ask your partner to tell you of any changes in the pain during treatment so you can determine which side is the better one to treat.

There are several areas of the ear that are helpful in all ear acupres-

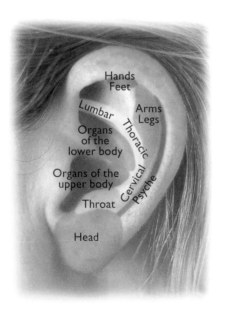

The most important regions of the body, as reflected in the ear. The white ring in the middle of the ear corresponds to areas of the spine. The lumbar spine is the lower back, the thoracic spine is the middle back, and the cervical spine is the upper back.

sure treatments—these include the general points, the antidepressant point, and the relaxation points. Treating these areas encourages general well-being for the body and mind. These points are discussed further under the therapies for specific ailments in the following chapter. See especially the Ear Acupressure sections on pages 33 and 35–36.

Ear acupressure can be performed with the recipient sitting up or lying down. Most of the time it's simpler to sit on a chair, because it's easier to move or to get up and walk around to determine if the ailing body part is feeling better. With a little practice, you will even be able to treat yourself.

Before beginning treatment, ask your partner to take conscious note of the location and intensity of his or her pain or other symptoms. Then, take your gem stick into your leading hand (usually the right hand), and gently but firmly hold the ear with the fingers of your left hand, making sure not to hurt your partner. Avoid pulling too hard on the ear, since this can cause pain in the middle ear.

Now think about the regions you want to treat, and slowly and gently stroke the tip of the stone over these spots. While doing this, pay attention to your partner's facial expression, and ask him or her to tell you when a spot is especially painful. If you are unable to find painful spots this way, apply a little more pressure to the potential areas on the ear with the tip of your stone. If your partner still does not register any pain, repeat the process with a little more pressure. Note that the earlobe is not as sensitive to pressure as is the rest of the ear structure.

Once you have located a painful point, remain on that spot with the tip of your massage stick for 10 to 20 seconds. Then remove the massage stick and ask your partner to move the ailing body part so you can assess the effects of therapy. If he or she notes significant or even a little improvement, you have found a good spot to treat. Return to this point, which will be easier to find now because the spot will show a small indentation and look redder than the surrounding skin. Touch the tip of your massage stick against the point again. It is okay if this feels somewhat unpleasant to your partner, as long as it is not painful. After another 10 to 20 seconds, again assess any change in your partner's

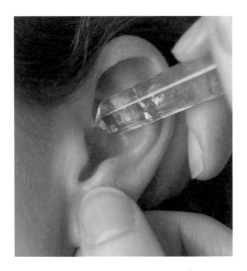

Hold the earlobe with your left hand and treat it with your right hand. (If you are left-handed, you may be more comfortable holding with your right hand and treating with your left.)

pain. If you do not record any further improvement, search the area surrounding the spot for other sensitive points. As long as you observe improvement after each treatment application, keep treating the same area until you note no further improvement.

If you encounter an initial worsening during a treatment application, do not be discouraged. The pain will eventually subside. However, you must be careful not to injure the skin, and always be sure that the discomfort on the ear is not too much for your partner. If your partner experiences a piercing pain while you are looking for sensitive spots, immediately remove the massage stick from the ear and ask your partner to lightly move the painful body part. It is possible that this short, hard treatment while searching may have been enough to relieve the pain. This is often the case with less serious ailments.

If you are treating an illness, such as a cough, as opposed to a painful joint or other body part, ask your partner between treatment applications whether his or her breathing has gotten easier or if the pressure in the chest has lessened. With some practice you will be able to see these changes in the recipient yourself: for example, when breathing becomes deeper, quieter, and more relaxed.

As long as you find and treat the right points, you will most likely notice improvement. Headaches are one exception; ear acupressure is not always helpful for headaches.

Cautions

Avoid infected or injured skin on the auricle (ear structure) during treatment. If you feel it is essential to treat such skin, do so only with extreme caution, making sure to avoid further damage.

For pregnant women, avoid treating the part of the ear that corresponds to the lower body during the first trimester (the first three months of pregnancy). Remember that treatment points are painful and be especially careful when searching for them on infants and small children. People who have epilepsy or other seizure disorders should receive treatment only from trained medical practitioners.

Body Acupressure

I use body acupressure techniques primarily to treat points on the face and hands. Finding the right body points to treat can be a difficult undertaking, especially since the corresponding body parts are not as well defined on the body as they are on the ear. It can take years of study to become proficient in locating body acupressure points. Practitioners who are very skilled and have been treating patients for many years may be able to feel the points that are in need of treatment because each point has a different skin resistance. However, a few select points on the body are well suited for the treatment of pain and illness and are also relatively easy to locate.

Application

To locate the body acupressure points discussed in this book, you will have to use the diagrams provided.

Treat the selected points using the tip of the gem stick, without massage oil. Apply the stone gently on the spot, but provide a steady pressure. Be patient, since each point must be treated for at least 5 minutes. As in ear acupressure, periodically ask your partner whether he or she notices any change or improvement in the pain. It is often helpful to combine body acupressure with another therapy such as ear acupressure or foot reflexology.

Cautions

Do not treat infected or injured skin or moles. Avoid pressing the tip of the gem stick deeply into the skin.

For infants and small children, a gentle touch will suffice. People who have epilepsy or other seizure disorders should receive treatment only from trained medical practitioners.

Foot Reflexology

In many cultures, including that of central Europe, foot reflexology remains an important part of traditional medicine. Details about this healing practice can be found in ancient records from all over the world. For example, records show that the Maya, who lived in and around the area that is now Mexico, used foot reflexology massages to treat a wide range of ailments.

If you have been to Thailand, you probably remember seeing many shops offering this type of treatment. To get the benefits of Thai foot reflexology, you need not even speak the language, because good therapists—often, young Thai women—can detect your ailments on the soles of your feet.

Just as in ear acupressure, in foot reflexology the parts of the foot that correspond to a sick organ are sensitive to pressure. In much the same way the body is reflected on the structure of the ear, the body is reflected on the sole of the foot. The head is located on the toes and areas of the back are found on the inner edge of the foot. The chest organs (the esophagus, trachea, bronchial tubes, lungs, heart, thymus, and diaphragm) are on the upper part of the sole near the ball of the foot. Farther down are the organs of the abdomen (the liver, gallbladder, stomach, spleen, pancreas, large and small intestines, and kidneys). Below that are the organs of the lower body, in particular the reproductive organs and bladder.

Organs that come in pairs (that is, the lungs, kidneys, adrenal glands, and some of the reproductive organs) are represented on both feet. All other organs are also represented on both feet, but more

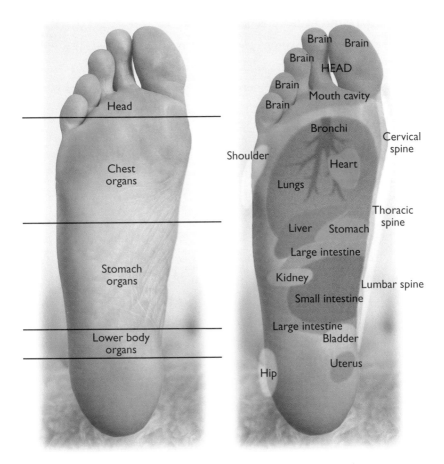

The regions of the body are reflected on the sole of the foot.

strongly on the side on which they are located. For example, the heart is reflected more strongly on the left foot, and the liver more on the right foot.

Application

Always treat both feet. If necessary, wash the feet before treatment with warm water. Wrap the foot that you are not working on in a warming towel. Do not use massage oil.

For the treatment, use the blunt end of the gem stick. First locate and massage (with the gem stick) any painful spots on the foot. For the therapy to be successful, it is not necessary to cause pain. Instead, be gentle, because foot reflexology should always support general well-being.

Before beginning treatment, ask the person you are treating to consciously feel his or her pain, just as you would for ear or body acupressure. This will allow you to gauge the success of your treatment.

First, take the foot you want to treat into your left hand and hold it steady. Now take the stone in your right hand and rub it across the sole of the foot with the blunt side. As you do this, carefully check the organ areas and note any sensitive spots. When you find a sensitive spot, massage it for a few seconds with the gem stick, using circular motions. If you encounter an initial worsening, which is rare, continue the treatment and the pain should quickly dissipate.

A holistic treatment (meaning a treatment that affects the whole body) should take about 30 minutes per foot and should be done on both feet. During the massage, ask your partner again to consciously feel his or her pain, asking whether there is any improvement or change in symptoms.

For acute ailments, perform treatment once or several times a day, or at least every other day. For chronic ailments, massage twice a week

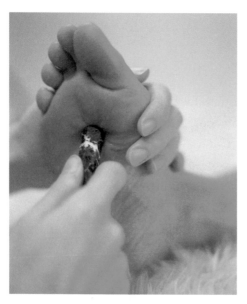

Use your left hand (or right if you are left-handed) to support and stabilize the foot during treatment. Hold the gem stick as you would a screwdriver.

for as long as necessary. With some practice and flexibility, self-treatment is possible.

A gentle massage revitalizes the body, whereas a strong one can cause the body to close up. Thus, if your partner suffers from constipation, you should massage very gently, with the goal of encouraging the activity of the intestines. (In such a case, it is also important to massage in the right direction; for more information, see Intestinal Cramps, Constipation, and Diarrhea, starting on page 84.)

After the massage, you can rub a pleasant massage oil on the feet, but if you do, make sure to allow enough time for the skin to absorb the oil before your partner must get up and walk around.

Cautions

Avoid injured or infected parts of the skin of the feet, including warts. Do not perform foot reflexology if the recipient has a fungal infection on his or her feet, because you could rub fungal spores deeper into the skin or spread the fungus to other parts of the body.

Be careful when treating pregnant women; do not massage the areas corresponding to the lower body during the first trimester (the first three months of pregnancy). People who have epilepsy or other seizure disorders should receive treatment only from trained medical practitioners.

Reflexology Massage

With gem massage sticks you can administer a number of different reflexology massages, usually focused on small regions of the body, such as the narrow area on either side of the spine. The positive energy of the gems plays an important role in the massage. Often, a simple gem stick reflexology massage can be sufficient to alleviate pain.

I find that reflexology massage is most effective when used in combination with ear acupressure, body acupressure, or foot reflexology techniques. For best results, begin the treatment session with ear acupressure or foot reflexology and finish with the reflexology massage. After reflexology massage, allow the recipient to rest quietly for about 30 minutes.

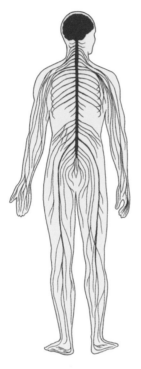

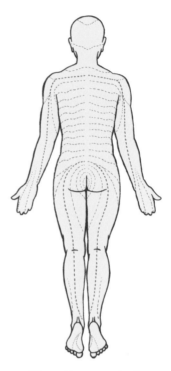

The main nerves of the peripheral nervous system, as seen from the back.

The reflex zones in the back are innervated by separate nerves.

I believe that every massage must be perceived as pleasant, although I know this contradicts the opinion of many other massage therapists. However, my success as a therapist has reinforced my belief that massage should not be painful. Even people who say they do not like massages because they are painful are happy to come back after they have experienced my gem stick massage techniques.

Reflexology massage is administered on the back, generally in a small area on either side of the spine. Properly applied, reflexology massage can have beneficial effects on the entire body, because the nerves that support the extremities (arms and legs) and many internal organs all originate in the spine. One such nerve is the sciatic nerve, which originates in the back but can cause pain extending from the lower back all the way down to the heels. Similarly, hip pains can originate in the back, and pain in the arms may originate in the neck. If you work seated at a desk all day, you may be all too familiar with these pains.

Each nerve originating from the spine innervates one part of the skin as well as the organs of the lower body regions, as shown in the diagram at left. These reflex zones are called Head zones in honor of British neurologist Sir Henry Head (1861–1940), who first discovered the correlation between the nerves in these skin zones and the internal organs.

When you stimulate the correct skin area with your gem stick, you stimulate the nerves and thus encourage the corresponding organ to heal itself. For example, regular reflexology massage of the correct skin zone can help improve digestion or alleviate an infection of the stomach lining.

Application

Apply massage oil to the back, and massage the selected areas using the blunt end of the gem stick. If you are not treating a specific pain or ailment, you can massage from the top down and back up again.

If the aim of the massage is to alleviate pain, the focus of the massage should be on the part of the spine that corresponds to the painful area. If the massage is intended to treat an ailment, you must treat the part of the spine that corresponds to the ailing area. For example, to help with heart ailments, you must massage the part of the spine that corresponds to the chest and heart (the thoracic spine area).

In the neck area (also known as the cervical spine area), you can massage up to the region just above the shoulders. In the thoracic spine area, massage only the region one to two inches on either side of the spine. You can massage a somewhat larger region in the lumbar spine area, a little lower down the back. In the sacral area, which is even farther down, again massage only a small area on either side of the spine. Do not massage the vertebrae themselves.

As mentioned previously, a basic principle of my treatment is that the massage must be perceived as pleasant. The duration of the massage will depend on the ailment, but a 20- to 30-minute treatment usually suffices.

Using your gem stick, massage in small circles or figure-eight patterns on the skin, applying a firm but gentle pressure. You can also brush from the spine outward with the stone. To do this, place the stone next to the spine and stroke outward, decreasing the pressure as you brush away from the spine. This movement can be likened to the technique used to produce a thick brushstroke in Chinese calligraphy.

Try out a few different techniques and ask your partner how he or she likes what you are doing. Let your imagination guide you. As long as you are massaging the muscle area near the spine and your partner is enjoying the sensation, you are doing the right thing.

Remember, the massage should never be painful. If necessary, reduce the pressure to gentle stroking along the back with the blunt end of the gem stick. The most important thing is to release the positive energy of the gem. In rare cases, gem sticks may amplify the pain. If such pain does not subside after a few minutes, end the massage.

Cautions

Avoid injured or infected skin, wounds, and moles during the massage. For pregnant women, do not treat the lumbar spine area during the first trimester (the first three months of pregnancy).

When working with very thin people, make sure that you do not massage the skin against protruding bones, vertebrae, or ribs. Be careful in general not to massage vertebrae or other bones, and be cautious with painful joints. People who have epilepsy or other seizure disorders should receive treatment only from trained medical practitioners.

Accompanying Holistic Therapies

Homeopathic and herbal remedies and other natural treatments can support acupressure and reflexology treatments in easing pain. It can also be beneficial to directly massage the part of the body that is in pain or even to just place the gemstone on the area.

For a massage, use the blunt end of the gem stick and some massage oil. Limit these massages to only a few minutes. Never massage a bone;

it would be too painful. You can massage the back to the left and right of the vertebrae. These massages should feel good. Make sure the recipient is kept comfortable and that the room is warm enough.

To place the gemstone on the painful place, use the long side of the gem stick and leave it there for about 30 minutes. While an initial worsening of pain during treatment is not uncommon, the pain should subside quickly. In rare cases, gem sticks can serve to amplify pain. If the pain does not subside after a few minutes, remove the stone.

If you have several gem sticks, you may want to try other stones on a problematic area. Try simply placing the blunt end of the stone against the spot and holding it there. The important thing here is not necessarily the touch, but rather the energy that emanates from the gemstone.

Massage Oil Recipes

Always use a good-quality massage oil. Many stores carry an excellent selection of massage oils, but you can also easily prepare your own blend at home.

If you have St. John's wort (*Hypericum perforatum*) in your garden, pick the flowers during the early summer, place them in a jar, and cover the blossoms with oil. Allow this to soak for at least two weeks and then strain the oil. Any good cold-pressed oil (except rapeseed oil) or jojoba oil is well suited for this purpose.

The following massage oil recipes are equally effective and can be prepared more quickly. Each recipe makes enough for one massage. Jojoba oil or any edible oil, such as sweet almond oil, is appropriate as a base oil for the other ingredients.

Salt Massage Oil
2 tablespoons jojoba or edible oil
$1/4$ teaspoon salt

Heat the oil in a water bath and dissolve the salt in the oil. You can prepare a larger quantity of this oil in advance and keep it in a glass bottle.

Relaxation Massage Oil

3 to 5 drops essential lavender oil

2 tablespoons jojoba or edible oil, such as almond oil

To make the massage oil, mix the essential oils into the base oil. Lavender has a calming effect and is good for the skin.

Muscle and Joint Massage Oil

10 drops rosemary essential oil

5 drops thyme essential oil

5 drops frankincense essential oil

2 tablespoons jojoba or edible oil, such as almond oil

To make the massage oil, mix the essential oils into the base oil. Rosemary and thyme essential oils stimulate good circulation, and frankincense has anti-inflammatory qualities.

Recuperation Massage Oil

1 to 2 drops rose essential oil, cubeb (*Litsea cubeba*)

essential oil, or another favorite essential oil

2 tablespoons jojoba or edible oil, such as almond oil

To make the massage oil, mix the essential oils into the base oil. With rose oil, which is very mild and gentle, you can indulge everyone. As a base oil, use jojoba oil, almond oil, or peanut oil, which have almost no scent of their own.

Choosing the Right Stone

There are a number of special techniques that can assist the practitioner in choosing the best gem stick for a specific person or application. The same methods—which include analytical kinesiology and hand rod and pendulum techniques—can also help you find the right areas and points to treat with body acupressure and reflexology.

However, if you do not know how to perform analytical kinesiology or use a hand rod or pendulum, you will still have good success with your treatments. Often enough, these measures simply serve to confirm that one is already on the right track. Even if none of your gem sticks seems optimally suited for a particular person or treatment, use them anyway. You may need to continue the treatment for a longer period of time, but the eventual treatment response will be much the same.

Analytical Kinesiology

Kinesiology is based on the principle that a negative (the "wrong" choice) will weaken muscle strength and a positive (the "right" choice) will strengthen the muscle. Performing kinesiology tests with gem sticks can help you determine which is the best stone to use in treating a particular individual. This requires a bit of practice and experience. However, if you have worked with kinesiology before, by all means try it with your gem sticks.

Ask the person you are treating to extend his or her right arm toward you. Take the wrist in your right hand and, while gently pressing downward, ask the person to resist your pressure. Take note of how much strength you can feel in your partner's arm. (If you are left-handed, use your left hand instead of the right.)

To see how this works, try the following test. To check that your partner's arm remains strong when receiving positive, correct information, take his or her arm, apply downward pressure, and ask silently whether your partner is male or female. If you receive the right answer and the muscle remains strong, you will know that the kinesiology test is working.

To determine which gemstone to use, place a stone against your partner's thymus (located near the heart) and silently ask, "Will this stone help?" Now check the muscle strength of the arm. If you have chosen the best stone, or even a good one, the muscle will remain strong.

One obstacle to success with this test is dehydration. If necessary, ask your partner to drink some water before performing the test.

Hand Rod or Pendulum

If you know how to use a hand rod or pendulum, you can easily find the gem stick best suited for treatment. Hold the rod in your right hand and silently tell the rod to go up and down to indicate a "yes" answer. The rod should go up and down. If that works, tell the rod to move left and right for "no." If the rod responds accordingly, take a gem stick in your left hand and ask "Will this gemstone help?" The rod will reflect what your subconscious can feel. The pendulum works in the same way. After instructing the pendulum how to move for both positive and negative answers, ask whether a particular gem will help while holding the gem stick in your hand opposite the pendulum. Since all stones have beneficial effects, waiting for an answer from a hand rod or pendulum is not critical to making a choice. Hand rods and pendulums can also be used to check that a particular gem stick is energetically clean and charged.

Finding the Right Spot to Treat

The basic principles for finding the correct areas and points to treat are the same as for finding the right stone. You may use analytical kinesiology or the hand rod or pendulum, just as you did for finding the right gem stick to use.

Note, however, that these techniques are not necessary for successful ear acupressure or foot reflexology, because spots requiring treatment will be painful to the touch and can be easily located simply by touching them with your gem stick.

Analytical Kinesiology

Place the gem stick you have chosen against the ailing body part or the selected acupressure point and ask if this is the right spot for treatment. You will know you are getting a positive response if the arm muscle remains strong.

You can even use this technique to check how long treatment should last. For example, you can ask, "Should the stone rest here for up to 5 minutes?" If the muscle remains weak, ask, "Up to 10 minutes?" Be sure to always include "up to" when you are trying to determine duration of treatment. That way if you inquire about 10 minutes and it is only 9 minutes 37 seconds, you will still receive a positive answer. When you have determined the correct length of time, you will know because the muscle will feel strong.

Hand Rod or Pendulum

For body acupressure and reflexology massage, you can use your hand rod or pendulum to find important spots to treat.

To do so, place the gem stick against the spot you think might need treatment. Hold the hand rod or pendulum in the other hand and ask if treatment of this spot will be beneficial. If you receive a positive answer, carry out the treatment as planned, continuing to hold the hand rod or pendulum. Wait until it comes to a resting place, at which point you will know the treatment of this spot is finished. I often work in this manner and am always pleased with the results. By now, I do not even need to ask questions, because the rod moves automatically to give me an answer. All I need to do is keep the rod near the patient.

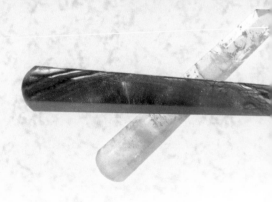

THERAPIES FROM
HEAD TO TOE

Acupressure and reflexology techniques play an important role in nearly all of my treatments. It is rare that a person suffers from one problem only, and it is possible to treat more than one ailment in one session. In such a case, choose one or two types of therapy and think about what exactly you want to treat before you begin. Mark the relevant pages in this book with Post-it notes or paper clips so that you can refer to them quickly to locate the correct points to treat. Don't forget to take this book and your gem stick with you when you travel.

It is always best to seek the advice of a trained health care practitioner to get a proper diagnosis for any serious health condition. However, many people who turn to me for help already have a long odyssey of medical treatment behind them and still do not have a definite diagnosis. Even though I may not be able to pinpoint the cause of their ailment myself, I can almost always alleviate or even heal it. If you have to wait for an appointment with your doctor, you may want to try treating yourself with your gem stick in the meantime. You may even find that your problem has disappeared by the time your appointment comes around.

If your specific health condition is not listed in this book, look for another ailment affecting the same organ or body part and carry out the treatment described there. As long as you do not cause injury with the gem stick—in other words, if you respect the rules about when not to use gem stick treatment—you can do no harm.

Skin

The skin is the largest organ of the body and has many vital functions. It is important to realize, however, that most skin problems originate inside the body. For example, neurodermatitis (a type of allergic dermatitis) is an illness of the immune system that affects the skin.

A good detoxification can be helpful in curing some skin problems, such as acne. However, because the exact origins of skin problems are often difficult to diagnose, most are quite difficult to treat.

Preferred stones: Fluorite and aventurine have beneficial effects for the skin. Rock crystal is effective in general against illness and infection. Heliotrope boosts the body's detoxification processes and immune defenses.

Ear Acupressure

While there are special skin points in the ear, treating them does not always produce noticeable effects. Experience shows that it makes more sense to treat all pressure-sensitive spots in the ear holistically. Chronic skin ailments should be treated two or three times a week, and acute ailments once or twice a day.

For chronic skin ailments, whether on one or several parts of the skin, you can stimulate the detoxification powers of the liver and kidneys by treating the spots in the ear that correspond to these organs. The skin ailment will improve only over time and after many treatments.

If you are treating an acute, localized skin condition or problem (for example, a scrape on the knee or a burn on the arm), simply treat the corresponding spots in the ear. Note that ear acupressure will not be effective against foot or nail fungal infections.

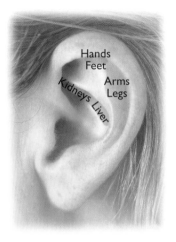

For chronic skin ailments, focus treatment on the internal organs. If needed, search the area of the arms and legs for painful spots.

Foot Reflexology

By treating the soles of the feet, you can stimulate the entire body's self-healing processes. As long as the skin ailment you are treating does not affect the soles of the feet, foot reflexology can be helpful. Again, the focus should be on stimulating the liver and kidneys to do their detoxification work. Treat both feet regularly over an extended period of time as necessary.

On the foot, locate and massage all pressure-sensitive spots. Also gently massage the spots corresponding to the liver and kidneys (see diagram on page 19).

Sadness, Stress, and Other Emotional Issues

Treatment with gem sticks is good for the spirit, whether one is experiencing depression, struggling with emotional stress or tension, or just feeling down. Regular gem stick treatment—meaning once or twice a week—can do wonders to stabilize the psyche, improving mood gently and without side effects.

Preferred stones: Rutile quartz is particularly helpful for depression and anxiety. Both rutile quartz and sodalite increase self-confidence. Rose quartz is considered one of the best stones for healing heartache and helping to release and process unexpressed emotions. Amethyst helps calm the nerves and promotes emotional centering; it is also help-ful for those trying to overcome addiction.

Ear Acupressure

There is a wonderful spot on the ear that helps with depression. This spot should be included in every ear acupressure treatment, and is pres-sure sensitive on almost all people. Of course this does not mean that all people suffer from depression, but a treatment that balances the psyche and brightens mood is something from which everyone can benefit.

The antidepressant point is located on the end of the ridge on the outer edge of the ear. Always treat both ears.

Treating this point does not usually lead to an immediate improve-ment, making it more difficult for you to verify the success of your treat-ment. Keep the tip of the massage stick on this pressure-sensitive spot for about 20 to 30 seconds.

Now move the tip upward along the ridge and treat any pressure-sensitive points you find for a few seconds each. This is simply good for the spirit. Along the middle of the ridge is a relaxation point that is particularly sensitive to pressure among most people. Treating this point helps calm and balance the psyche.

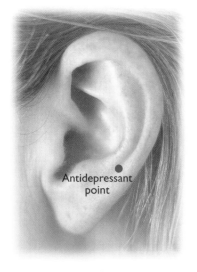

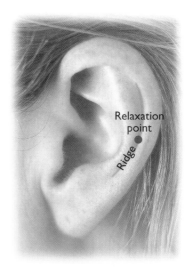

Reflexology Massage

A gentle gem stick massage of all reflex zones on the back with scented massage oil often accomplishes miracles for those suffering from emotional distress. Always perform this treatment after ear acupressure.

Since the neck muscles are often tense during times of psychological stress, the focus of the massage treatment should be on the neck and shoulder area. Put on some soothing music for the massage. After about 20 minutes of treatment, allow the recipient to rest for 20 minutes. Cover him or her with a blanket or a towel during this rest period.

Treating the neck and shoulder area is good for the soul. Even simply placing a hand here helps the recipient feel better. Think of the expres-

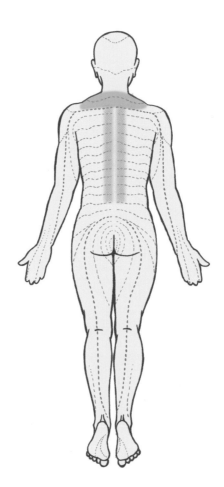

sion "shouldering a heavy burden" and you will understand how important the neck and shoulder area can be in cases of emotional distress.

Accompanying Holistic Therapies

A good homeopathic remedy for sadness is Ignatia LM6. If needed, take 3 to 5 pellets two or three times a day for a few days.

St. John's wort is an herbal remedy that can be effective against depression. For best results, it should be taken for at least several weeks at a time, either as a tea or in the form of capsules or tablets. Effects become apparent only after about three weeks. If you are taking any pharmaceutical medications, discuss the use of St. John's wort with your doctor first.

Sleep Problems

Sleep disorders, such as insomnia, can have a variety of causes, including external disturbances. A digital radio alarm clock or halogen lamp near the bed creates electric pollution that can disrupt sleep. The first thing to do is remove these external influences.

Also, consider the beverages you are drinking during the day and before bedtime. Avoid caffeine, which is found in coffee, chocolate, colas, and tea, even green tea. I often encounter people who do not know that green tea is a strong stimulant. In addition, don't drink too much liquid just before bedtime, so you won't wake up in the middle of the night needing to use the bathroom.

Preferred stones: Amethyst, aventurine, and heliotrope help against internal unrest, and amethyst can be particularly helpful for insomnia. Sodalite also encourages sleep.

Ear Acupressure

First locate and treat both general ear points. One of these is located at the tip of the triangle in the upper part of the ear, the other on the center axis of the ear. Also treat the antidepressant point.

Aside from the general relaxation point in the ridge of the ear,

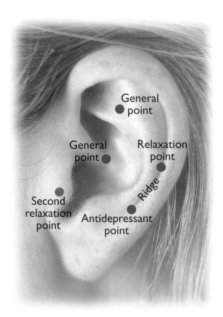

another important point can be found on the opposite side of the ear. The entire ridge and each of these points should be treated for about 5 minutes every night before you go to bed.

Reflexology Massage

Perform this massage at night, while your partner is in bed preparing to fall asleep. Use a lavender massage oil, because lavender has calming effects.

Gently massage the whole area to the right and left of the upper spine with the blunt end of the gem stick. It is important that your massage technique is soothing and not too stimulating. However, it is not just the massage technique but also the attention at nighttime that can work miracles, especially with children.

Massaging the lower half of the body may overstimulate the kidneys, with the possibility that your partner will wake up shortly after falling asleep because he or she has to use the bathroom.

Accompanying Holistic Therapies

To return to a regular sleeping rhythm, it can be helpful to take valerian, lemon balm (melissa), or hops as a tea, tincture, or capsule at nighttime.

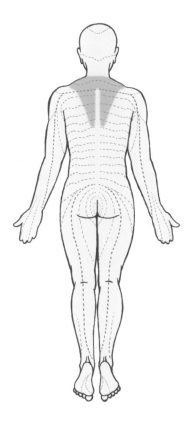

Follow the manufacturer's dosage recommendations. In some cases, especially with children, placing 1 to 3 drops of lavender oil on the pillow can help induce sleep.

Concentration Difficulties

Many people have difficulty keeping their mind on things. This condition is easy to see in children—they lose interest in a game after a few minutes or continually ask for new sheets of paper when drawing. They lack the patience to remain focused on one task, which can have detrimental effects on their school performance and other aspects of their lives.

In extreme cases, such people are unable to learn and work with an appropriate amount of concentration. Regular acupressure can provide at least some relief from the problem.

Preferred stones: Fluorite is good for concentration. Rock crystal provides energy and clarity, while amethyst emanates calm. Rutile quartz offers stability.

Ear Acupressure

Concentration ability is linked to brain function, so check the head area of the ear (the earlobe) for painful spots. Immediate improvement of the condition will not be noticeable; thus, you should treat all painful spots for about 20 to 30 seconds each.

Be sure to check the points that have effects on the psyche, which are located along the ridge of the ear. All points that are noticeable here should be treated briefly. Also locate and treat both general ear points. One is located at the tip of the triangle in the upper ear, the other on the center axis of the ear.

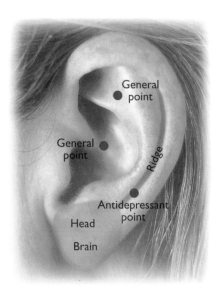

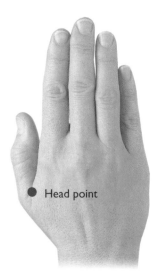

Body Acupressure

On both hands, there is a point that has beneficial effects for brain function.

Place your thumb on the hand, turn the back of the hand toward you, and steady the recipient's hand using your free hand. There is a fold of skin between the thumb and the hand at the end of which, on the highest spot, is a point that you initially simply should touch with the pointed edge of your gem stick. Now have the recipient relax his or her hand and remain on this spot with your stone for 2 to 3 minutes. Treat both hands in this manner.

Accompanying Holistic Therapies

Placing 1 or 2 drops of cubeb (*Litsea cubeba*) or lemongrass (*Cymbopogon citratus*) essential oils on the collar or in an oil lamp can encourage concentration.

Concentration problems can be caused by a lack of vitamins, best remedied by eating a good diet and taking a multivitamin and mineral preparation.

Headache and Migraine

Headaches cannot always be treated with gem sticks, because the cause of pain in the head is rarely inside the head itself. Nevertheless, do try to help the patient.

If the cause of headache pain is a sinus infection or neck tension, however, ear acupressure is often highly effective. In cases of migraine, it may at least be possible to alleviate nausea. Over the long term, treating the ear or the sole of the foot as part of a holistic treatment plan may also help with migraine.

Sometimes headaches are caused by a lack of vitamins, hormonal imbalances, a bad diet, or allergies. Keeping a headache or migraine diary can help the sufferer pinpoint factors that trigger pain or migraine attacks.

Preferred stones: Amethyst is effective against tension and weak nerves and helps alleviate pain, much as aventurine does. Aventurine is particularly helpful against migraine. Rock crystal is good in general against illnesses, and sodalite strengthens the nerves. Rose quartz has a positive influence on female hormones.

Ear Acupressure

First locate the two general points and treat for about 20 seconds with the pointed end of your gem stick. One is located at the tip of the triangle in

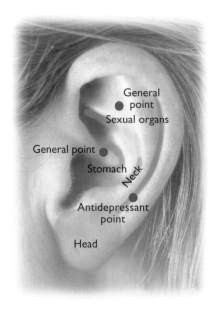

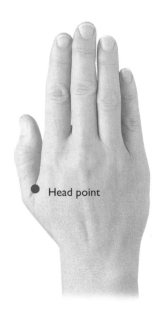

the upper part of the ear, the other on the center axis of the ear. Treating the antidepressant point and points along the ridge of the ear, for 10 to 20 seconds each, can also be helpful.

If the recipient's headache is caused by neck tension, treat the area of the ear that corresponds to the neck. Interestingly, it is located immediately adjacent to the antidepressant point. To be most effective, search this entire area for painful spots; you may find two or three. Treat these spots and then ask your partner whether or not the headache has decreased.

Deeper in the ear, you will find the stomach area. If your partner is experiencing nausea due to migraine, search in this area for points and treat any painful ones for 10 to 20 seconds.

Finally, search the earlobe (the head area) for sensitive points. This will be especially effective for a headache caused by a cold or a sinus infection.

If the headache has hormonal causes, also treat the area of the reproductive organs two or three times a week over several months.

Body Acupressure

There is an important point on the hands for headaches, and it can be used for self-treatment as well as for treating a partner. This is a relatively large acupressure point. To locate it, have your partner extend his or her hand with the thumb resting against the fingers. This creates an elevated spot on the fold between the thumb and the hand, and at its highest point you will find the correct spot.

Initially, steady your partner's hand and simply touch the spot gently with the tip of your gem stick. Then ask your partner to relax his or her hand and keep the tip of the gem stick on the spot for 2 to 3 minutes. Be sure to treat both hands. Between applications, ask your partner whether the headache is getting better.

Foot Reflexology

The head is represented on the toes of both feet. Touch each toe individually, and then massage all of the toes for 1 to 2 minutes each with the blunt end of the gem stick. Since the treatment is intended to calm the pain, you should apply slightly stronger pressure. Unfortunately, the toes tend to be so small that treating the head area can be difficult.

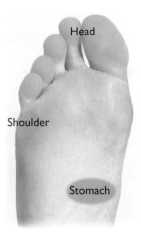

In the case of nausea, search the upper middle area of the sole of the foot for painful spots. If needed, massage the whole area with the gem stick in circular motions for 2 to 3 minutes.

For those who have frequent headaches or migraine attacks, regular holistic treatment can be helpful. This means examining the soles of the feet for painful spots two or three times a week and massaging the spots with the gem stick for about 30 minutes.

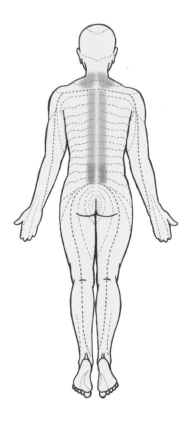

Reflexology Massage

When treating headache, reflexology massage, using the blunt end of the gem stick, is an excellent accompaniment to ear acupressure and should be performed after the ear treatment.

If the headache is related to muscle tension, massaging the neck can be very relaxing. If the cause is hormonal—for example, when headaches appear to be linked to menstruation—massage the lumbar vertebra area two or three times a week. Massaging the entire back to the right and left of the spine is an important part of holistic treatment. This should be done on a regular basis as needed.

Accompanying Holistic Therapies

Applying 1 or 2 drops of pure peppermint essential oil to the forehead can be beneficial against headache, especially if you apply it at the onset of the headache.

Peppermint or ginger tea can help with nausea. To make ginger tea, grate a small piece of fresh ginger and add hot water. If you suspect vitamin deficiency, a good multivitamin and mineral supplement is essential.

Earache

Earaches have various causes, but all of them are located in the head. Thus, the best approach is to treat the head area on the sole of the foot or on the ear. All reflexology and acupressure techniques can be combined to good effect.

Earaches may be caused by middle ear infection, sinus suppuration, or even a severe cold. Many earaches occur when the eustachian tube (the connecting tunnel between the middle ear and the nose) becomes blocked, which leads to painful pressure in the middle ear. When you treat the entire head area, you will be treating the cause (the illness) and the pain at the same time.

In rare cases, ear pain is due to excessive earwax. When there is a mechanical problem like this, gem stick treatment will not be successful. The earwax must be removed.

Preferred stones: Amethyst alleviates pain. Rock crystal reduces swelling and inflammation and helps in general with illnesses. Fluorite has beneficial effects on mucous membranes. You can also use heliotrope to boost the body's immune defenses.

Ear Acupressure

First locate and treat both general ear points. One is located at the tip of the triangle in the upper part of the ear, and the other one is on the center axis.

Since the ears are a part of the head, you should locate and treat painful spots in the head area of the ear (the earlobe). You will probably encounter painful spots on the affected side. However, the earlobe is less sensitive to pain than other parts of the ear, making it a little more difficult to locate spots to be treated. During acupressure, avoid

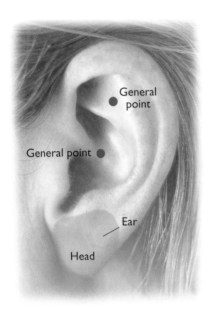

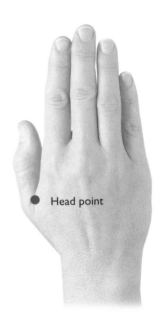

pulling on the ear, since this can increase the pain in the middle ear.

If the cause of the earache is a cold, treat the earlobes of both ears.

Body Acupressure

On the hand is a point that should be treated for all ailments in the head area, including earaches. To locate this point, have your partner extend his or her hand with the thumb resting against the fingers. This creates an elevated spot.

With your free hand, support the hand to be treated and place the tip of the gem stick on the highest spot. Now have your partner relax his or her hand. Press the tip of the stone on this relatively large acupressure point for 2 to 5 minutes.

Foot Reflexology

On the sole of the foot, just below the second smallest toe, is a spot that corresponds to the ear. Place the blunt end of the gem stick on this spot for 5 to 10 minutes. While doing this, move the stone in a slightly circular fashion.

In keeping with a holistic approach, massage all pressure-sensitive spots on both feet with the blunt end of the gem stick.

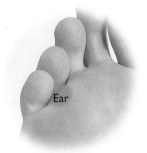

Accompanying Holistic Therapies

A warm chamomile poultice or salt bag placed on the ear will help alleviate pain. In addition, 3 pellets of the homeopathic remedy Belladonna D12 can be taken three times a day while symptoms persist.

Colds and Sinus Infections

Acupressure and reflexology can help even with severe colds and sinus problems. If the person responds to these therapies, a few intensive treatment sessions are usually sufficient to alleviate the ailment.

Because the trigeminal nerve runs along the face in close proximity to the sinuses, trigeminal neuralgia can be treated in the same way.

Preferred stones: Heliotrope increases the body's immune defenses. Aventurine is helpful against sinus problems. Fluorite has beneficial effects on the mucous membranes and is especially effective against infections of the respiratory tract. Rock crystal is helpful in general against illnesses and reduces inflammation.

Ear Acupressure

Ear acupressure is ideal for treating colds and sinus infections. First locate and treat the two general points in the ear. One is located at the tip of the triangle in the upper part of the ear, the other on the center axis of the ear.

Next, search the entire head area (the earlobe) for sensitive spots. Treat each of these for 20 to 30 seconds using the tip of the gem stick. Ask your partner in between treatment applications whether the congestion is

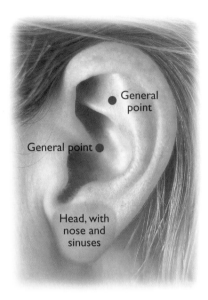

getting better. Be sure to follow this treatment with body acupressure on the face and hands.

Body Acupressure

The most important points for colds and sinus infections are easily found on the face. They are particularly easy to find because they are located to the left and right of the nose and above the eyebrows. The lower points can be very sensitive, so be careful in this area. Treatment should not be painful; the energy of the gem stick should be sufficient to provide a healing effect.

There are two spots next to the nose that you may be able to feel with your fingers. You will notice small indentations—to be more specific, holes—in the bones of this area. The trigeminal nerve runs through these holes. It innervates the whole area that you should treat. Thus, it is sufficient to place the tip of the gem stick against these spots for 30 seconds each, making sure to avoid pressing too hard.

Place the blunt end of the stone against the point between the eyebrows and the two points above the eyebrows. Hold the gem stick on each point for 30 seconds.

Also treat the head point on both hands. To locate this relatively large

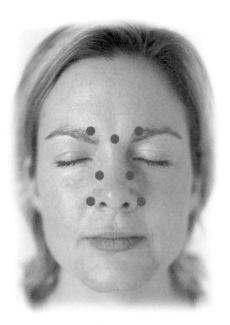

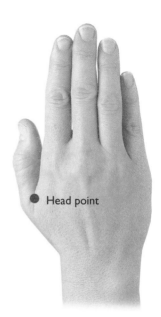

Head point

acupressure point, have your partner extend his or her hand with the thumb resting against the fingers. This creates an elevated spot on the fold between the thumb and the hand, and at its highest point you will find the correct spot. Support the hand to be treated with your left hand and place the tip of the gem stick on the elevated part. Ask your partner to relax his or her hand, and leave the gem stick on this spot for 2 to 5 minutes.

Foot Reflexology

The head and sinuses are represented on the bottom of the toes of both feet. Touch each toe individually and massage each one with the blunt end of the gem stick for 1 to 2 minutes. Unfortunately, the toes

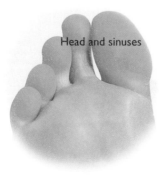

Head and sinuses

are usually so small that it is difficult to treat the head area effectively in this way.

In keeping with a holistic approach, it can be helpful to use your gem stick to massage the whole body on both soles of the feet.

Accompanying Holistic Therapies

Thyme tea helps with congestion and can be taken by adults or children three times a day.

The homeopathic medicine Luffa D4 is another remedy that can be effective against congestion. The dosage is 3 pellets several times a day.

Toothache

If you develop a toothache, you should of course see your dentist. However, acupressure can help alleviate the pain in the meantime.

After a dental treatment, nerves in the teeth may be irritated and painful. A treatment with the gem stick can be helpful in such instances (for example, after having a tooth pulled). Perform ear acupressure followed by body acupressure on the hands for best results.

Preferred stones: Amethyst and aventurine alleviate pain. Rock crystal helps against swelling and inflammation after dental treatment.

Ear Acupressure

Since the teeth are part of the head, locate and treat the area of the ear that corresponds to the head area (that is, the earlobe). The earlobe is less sensitive to pressure than the rest of the ear, making it slightly more difficult to locate the right spots.

To help ease fear before a dental procedure, treat the relaxation point on the ridge near the edge of the ear and the two general points. One of these is located at the tip of the triangle in the upper ear, the other on the center axis of the ear.

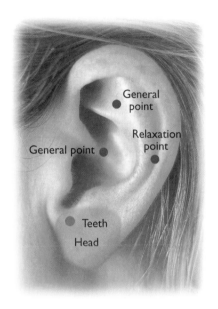
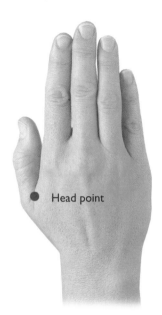

Body Acupressure

Toothaches on the right side of the mouth are treated on the right hand and vice versa. Only in rare cases will sensitive spots be found on the side opposite the problem area.

On the hand is a point that should be treated for all ailments in the head area, including toothaches. To locate this relatively large acupressure point, ask your partner to extend his or her hand with the thumb resting against the fingers. This creates an elevated spot on the fold between the thumb and the hand, and at its highest point you will find the correct spot.

Use your free hand to support the hand to be treated and place the tip of the gem stick on the highest point. Now ask your partner to relax his or her hand, and leave the gem stick on this spot for 2 to 5 minutes.

You can make your own visit to the dentist more bearable by keeping your gem stick on this spot during the dental procedure. If the teeth being treated are in the front of the mouth, alternately treat both hands.

Foot Reflexology

Locate the head and teeth on the sole of the foot on the painful side (the side of the body on which you have a toothache). The point to massage

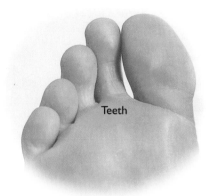

is at the top of the sole, just below the middle toes. Support the foot with one hand and locate and massage the painful spot for 1 to 2 minutes with the blunt end of the gem stick.

Accompanying Holistic Therapies

Before and after a dental procedure, take the homeopathic medication Arnica D12. Take 3 pellets immediately before the treatment; afterward, take 3 pellets every 30 minutes until pain and swelling subside.

Sore Throat

Colds often begin with a sore throat. Thus, it makes sense to treat the nose, lungs, and bronchial tubes all at the same time. It is a good idea to also immediately begin taking the accompanying holistic therapies listed below as soon as you notice you have a sore throat, to help prevent the development of a more serious infection.

Preferred stones: Sodalite has beneficial effects for the throat, fluorite for the mucous membranes. Rock crystal helps against inflammation and illness in general. Heliotrope boosts the body's immune system defenses.

Ear Acupressure

First locate and treat the two general points in the ear. One is located at the tip of the triangle in the upper part of the ear, the other on the center axis of the ear.

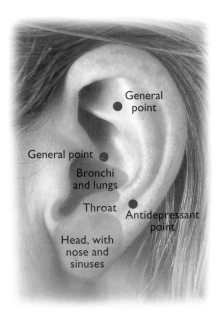

The throat points are located on the earlobe, on the edge of the deeper part of the auricle (the external ear structure). Locating and massaging these points require some skill, since the edge of the ear itself will be painful. As you search for and treat points, remember to ask your partner intermittently whether his or her swallowing has become easier.

To either prevent or alleviate a cold or flu, search the entire earlobe for painful spots and treat any that you find. The areas corresponding to the bronchi and lungs tend to be more sensitive in general, so touch these areas gently. For best results, use a gentle approach during this entire acupressure treatment. Treat each point for 20 to 30 seconds. The whole treatment can take up to 30 minutes.

To conclude, treat the antidepressant point for 20 to 30 seconds.

Foot Reflexology

The throat area is located at the top of both soles, just below the toes. Search for painful spots in this area and massage any that you find with the blunt end of the stick for 1 to 2 minutes.

In the spirit of holistic therapy, it can be helpful to massage the whole body via the foot, especially the bronchial tube and lung areas located slightly farther down the soles of both feet (see illustration on page 69).

Accompanying Holistic Therapies

Gargle with sage tea. In addition, especially when a sore throat develops into bronchitis or a cold, drinking 3 cups of thyme tea a day can help.

Neck Tension and Pain

Neck tension and pain afflict many people, and I am delighted time and again to see how effective ear acupressure is in alleviating these ailments, even if they have existed for a long time. For best results, follow ear acupressure with a massage of the neck area.

Neck pain may be felt as a burning sensation in the muscles. Often, the sufferer will be unable to turn his or her head in both directions in a normal manner. Even the range of motion of the arms can be affected. Sometimes the pain will extend down to the pinkie finger, or the fingers will tingle or become numb.

Preferred stones: Amethyst and aventurine are effective for tension and pain. Rock crystal is helpful against paralysis, and rose quartz encourages good blood circulation.

Ear Acupressure

First locate and treat the two general points in the ear. One of these is located at the tip of the triangle in the upper part of the ear, the other on the center axis of the ear. It can be helpful also to treat the antidepressant point, found at the end of the ridge at the edge of the ear.

However, the most important points are located next to the spine area. Look carefully for painful spots; there may be only a single one. To make sure you know which point is effective, ask your partner to pull up his or her shoulders after the treatment of each painful spot you've identified. Sometimes the burning pain will fade immediately, and it is important you know as soon as this happens.

If the cervical spine is the source of the neck problem, it must be included in the treatment. This requires some skill and practice, since the cervical spine area is located very near the neck area, on the inner edge of the ear. Have your partner turn his or her head sideways between treatments, so you can see if the range of motion has improved.

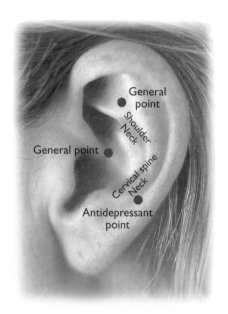

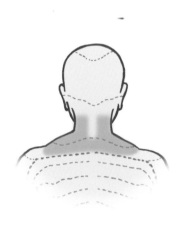

Accompanying Holistic Therapies

Perform a gem stick massage of the affected area after the ear acupressure treatment, using muscle and joint massage oil. Do not massage too firmly, because this can lead to muscle soreness. The energy of the stone and the healing effect of the massage oil will suffice to stimulate the body's self-healing powers. Regular treatment is generally more effective than a single, intensive massage.

The massage should take between 15 and 20 minutes. Afterward, while your partner is resting, place a warm grain pillow or cherry pit pillow on his or her neck.

Shoulder and Arm Pain

Shoulder pain often extends down to the arm. The sufferer may receive a diagnosis of "shoulder-arm syndrome," a term indicating that the true cause of the pain is unclear. Nerve infections can be particularly painful; an infection in the upper arm can cause pain all the way down to the fingertips. Arthrosis (degenerative joint disease) is rarely the cause of such shoulder and arm problems.

Regular acupressure treatments can help, whether the cause of the pain is known or unknown. Ear acupressure is probably more effective than foot reflexology for this problem. Because the cause of pain plays only a minor role in acupressure treatment, gem stick treatment can do wonders here to reduce pain and stimulate healing. Follow ear acupressure or foot reflexology with a reflexology massage using muscle and joint massage oil.

You must be very careful and gentle when treating the actual painful areas with the gem stick. Sometimes it suffices to simply place the stone lengthwise on the most severely affected area and leave it there for 30 minutes. Such an area should be massaged only very gently, using the blunt side of the stone. Do not massage the area if the cause of the pain is a nerve infection. In such a case, massage would only further irritate the nerves.

Preferred stones: Aventurine and amethyst alleviate pain and tension. Rock crystal is helpful against paralysis. Rose quartz and heliotrope stimulate good blood circulation. In the case of nerve infections, amethyst and sodalite can be beneficial.

Ear Acupressure

Ear acupressure is the preferred treatment for shoulder and arm pain. Be sure to treat both ears, but focus on the affected side.

The shoulder is reflected on two spots in the ear. Both are near the spine area. If there is pain in the neck that extends down to the shoulder, treat the neck area in the ear as well. However, the cause of the pain may be in the shoulder itself. Before the treatment, determine the degree of pain and your partner's range of motion. Then locate the most important shoulder points in the ear, next to the spine area, and treat these. In between treatment applications, gauge the success of your treatment by asking your partner to move his or her shoulder and arm.

With some patients, I have located painful spots a little deeper in the ear, in the area that corresponds to the lungs. Thus it makes sense to check this area for painful spots as well. Judging your partner's range of movement will enable you to determine quickly whether there are spots that need treatment in this area.

After about 15 minutes of treatment, you should be able to observe improvement. Chronic illnesses, including calcium deposits, should be treated two or three times a week with ear acupressure.

Foot Reflexology

The shoulder area is easy to find on the sole of the foot, because it is located just below the pinkie toe. Using the blunt end of the gem stick, massage this spot on both feet, focusing on the affected side. In between massage treatments, ask your partner to move his or her shoulder so you can gauge the success of the therapy.

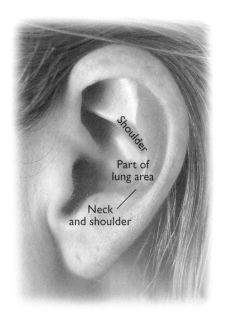

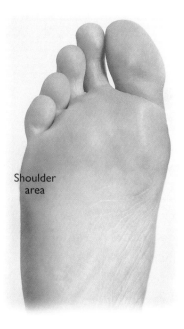

Reflexology Massage

Perform this massage after ear acupressure or foot reflexology. Massage only the areas to the right and left of the upper thoracic spine area. This is where the nerve endings for the shoulders are located.

Use muscle and joint massage oil for this massage. After applying the oil to the area, including the shoulders, massage only the small area on both sides of the spine for 10 to 15 minutes, using the blunt end of the gem stick.

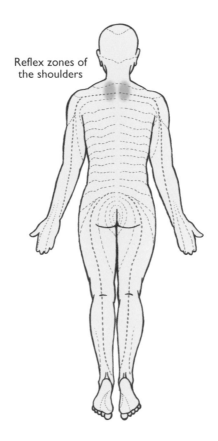

Reflex zones of the shoulders

Accompanying Holistic Therapies

In most cases, a warming pillow provides a pleasant sensation. Applying a magnet "Band-Aid" on the painful areas for a few days may further alleviate the pain. Supplement with vitamins B_1 and B_6 in cases of nerve infection.

Elbow Pain

Pain in the elbow is usually caused by infection or inflammation of the bursa or tendon sheath. "Tennis elbow," for example, known in medical terminology as bursitis, is an inflammation of the bursa (the sac that separates the tendon from the bone). Ear acupressure can be helpful in relieving this and other types of elbow pain.

Exercise great caution when massaging around the elbow joint. Do not massage protruding bones. You can massage the muscles of the upper and lower arm using the blunt side of the gem stick, as long as your partner perceives this as a pleasant sensation.

Preferred stones: Amethyst alleviates pain, and rock crystal reduces inflammation. Rose quartz and heliotrope encourage good blood circulation.

Ear Acupressure

Unfortunately, the elbow area is difficult to find inside the ear, because the exact location is different for every person. Thus, for the first treatment, you will probably have to search around a relatively large area (see diagram on page 58). The ear on the unaffected side requires only a brief treatment.

Once you have found and treated the painful spots, ask your partner to move his or her elbow. If the pain subsides while you are on a certain point, keep the gem stick there for a while. Ask your partner to report any reduction in the intensity of the pain while you are doing this. If you find a good point, remain on this spot with the gem stick until the pain in the elbow is alleviated.

During subsequent treatments, you should have an easier time locating the spots to treat. Most elbow problems must be treated several times. For best results, perform the treatment two or three times a week.

Reflexology Massage

The nerves that innervate the arms, including the elbows, are located to the right and left of the lower part of the cervical spine and upper

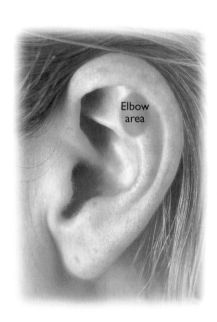

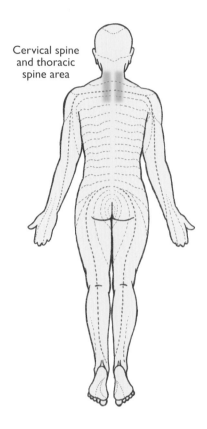

Cervical spine and thoracic spine area

Elbow area

thoracic spine. The lowest cervical vertebra is easy to recognize, since it protrudes slightly and does not move when the head is turned.

Massage this area using muscle and joint massage oil and the blunt end of the gem stick. You can massage a slightly larger area if the neck muscles are also tense. Only in rare cases will you see an immediate improvement after reflexology massage, but massage does help support the effects of ear acupressure.

Accompanying Holistic Therapies

Rub the elbow joint two or three times a day with muscle and joint massage oil. If the pain is due to an injury, such as falling on the elbow or lower arm, take 3 pellets of the homeopathic remedy Arnica D6 or D12 every hour.

Wrist Pain

Wrists are under a lot of stress, since all of us work with our hands to some extent. In addition, when we fall, we invariably try to protect the head and the rest of the body by extending our arms and falling directly onto the wrists. The wrists and lower arms are thus especially vulnerable to sprains and fractures.

Regardless of the source of the pain, ear acupressure will help to alleviate pain and support the healing process. (For pain related to carpal tunnel syndrome, see Finger and Thumb Pain, page 61.)

Preferred stones: Rock crystal helps reduce swelling and increase joint mobility. Amethyst alleviates pain. Rose quartz and heliotrope both support good blood circulation.

Ear Acupressure

The correct points are usually easy to locate, because they are all grouped in a small area in the upper part of the ear. Once you have found and briefly treated a sensitive spot, ask your partner to move his or her wrist as you hold the gem stick on the point. If you have found a good spot, the pain will immediately subside. Locate points in this area and treat until you notice no further improvement when your partner moves his or her wrist.

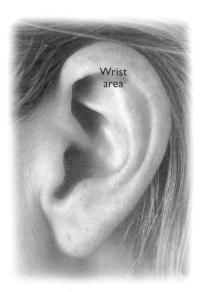

Wrist
area

For acute problems, a few treatments should suffice. Chronic wrist pain should be treated several times a week over an extended period of time until the pain is alleviated.

Reflexology Massage

Reflexology massage may be effective only for chronic wrist ailments. The nerves of the lower arms and wrists originate from the lower part of the cervical spine and the upper part of the thoracic spine. Accordingly, you should massage the whole area to the right and left of the spine. The lowest cervical vertebra is easy to recognize, since it protrudes and does not move when the head is turned. If you choose to administer this massage, perform it after the ear acupressure treatment.

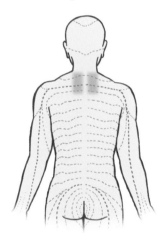

Accompanying Holistic Therapies

If you choose to massage the painful area of the wrist itself, be careful when massaging very thin people, as it is possible to rub the bones too vigorously during a localized massage. However, if there is a layer of muscle or fat to protect the bones, you can gently massage the affected areas using the blunt end of the gem stick, as long as this does not worsen the symptoms.

Rub the wrists two or three times a day with muscle and joint massage oil. If the pain is due to an acute injury, such as falling on the hands, take 3 pellets of the homeopathic remedy Arnica D6 or D12 every hour.

Finger and Thumb Pain

Finger and thumb pain is often caused by arthritis. While ear acupressure can be very helpful, a single treatment rarely suffices. For best results with chronic pain, regular treatment is necessary. Ear acupressure can also help with acute pain, such as the pain of a bruised, cut, or burned finger.

Pain or numbness in a part of the finger, especially if it occurs at night, may be caused by carpal tunnel syndrome. This problem may be related to the existence of a "tight spot" in the wrist caused by growths or deposits, which can pinch the nerves and lead to problems. Regular acupressure treatment of the wrist can help alleviate pain, especially if treatment is undertaken early on, when the problem first emerges.

Preferred stones: Rock crystal helps reduce swelling and inflammation and improves joint mobility. Amethyst alleviates pain, and rose quartz encourages good blood circulation. Fluorite helps with pain related to arthritis.

Ear Acupressure

Finding the finger area in the ear is not difficult, because the fingers are reflected at the very top of the ear. As with other joint ailments, ask your partner to move his or her fingers before and during the treatment so you can evaluate the success of the therapy. (With acute

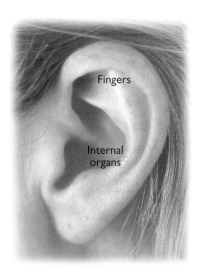

problems, your partner will notice an improvement without moving the fingers.)

For chronic ailments, you will achieve best results if you perform the treatment regularly (two or three times a week). If you are treating arthritis, a holistic approach will be helpful. Thus, locate and treat all sensitive spots in the area of the ear corresponding to the internal organs.

For acute pain, simply perform ear acupressure treatment as needed.

Foot Reflexology

In keeping with a holistic approach, using the blunt end of the gem stick to massage the whole body on both soles of the feet can be very helpful. Be on the lookout for pain-sensitive spots.

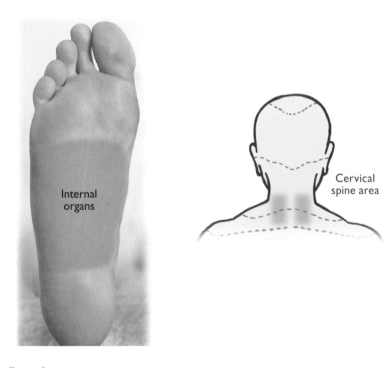

Reflexology Massage

Reflexology massage can help alleviate pain in the fingers only for chronic conditions. If you choose to carry out this gem stick massage, perform it after ear acupressure.

Most of the nerves for the fingers originate in the lower part of the cervical spine. Massage only this small area to the right and the left of the spine. The lowest cervical vertebra is easy to recognize because it protrudes slightly and does not move when the head is turned.

Accompanying Holistic Therapies

Apply muscle and joint massage oil to the affected parts two or three times a day.

Back Pain

Low back pain is very common, and many therapists make their living treating only this problem. A good ear or foot acupressure treatment, perhaps combined with a reflexology massage, can significantly reduce back pain or even relieve it altogether.

Preferred stones: Aventurine and amethyst alleviate pain and tension. Rock crystal reduces swelling and helps with paralysis. Rose quartz and heliotrope encourage good blood circulation. Sodalite has positive effects on the nerves.

Ear Acupressure

First locate and treat the two general points in the ear. One of these is located at the tip of the triangle in the upper part of the ear, the other on the center axis of the ear.

Treating the area in the ear that corresponds to the spine requires some skill and practice. However, this is not as important as treating the adjoining areas that represent the back muscles. The areas of the ear that correspond to these muscles are located to the right and left of the spine areas in the ear.

Treating the area that corresponds to the back muscles is easy, except when it comes to the very end of the spine, the sacral area. It is difficult to reach under the rim of the ear with the stone. If you do not understand what I mean, look at the back line of an actual ear, and you will see that the line extends all the way to the wall of the ear, close to the

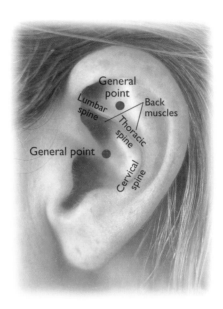

skull. However, you will have to treat this area extensively only if the pain is felt in the very lowest part of the back, almost on the buttocks. If necessary, you can gently treat this area using a paper clip bent into an open position.

The spine itself is represented directly on the inner ridge of the ear. Performing acupressure in this area requires some skill, but you will not cause any harm if you treat the wrong parts, so feel free to experiment and practice. The higher up on the back the pain is felt, the farther down the ear ridge the main points will be.

Ask your partner to move every once in a while or even get up and walk around in order to verify the results of your treatment. You may want to treat your partner in a seated position instead of lying down, so that it is easier for him or her to get up during treatment. If you note a significant improvement after treating a certain point, continue treating this spot until no further improvement occurs.

For acute pain, perform ear acupressure up to three times a day. For chronic back pain, treat once or twice a week over an extended period of time.

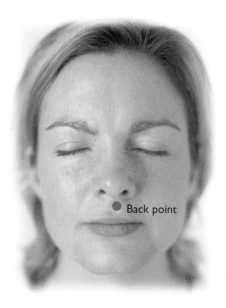

Back point

Body Acupressure

There are many points on the body that are good for back pain. Locating the right points can be difficult for a novice. However, if the pain is in the lumbar area, there is an effective point on the face that is very easy to locate, since it is precisely between the nose and the upper lip. Treat this point for 2 to 3 minutes with the pointed end of the gem stick.

Ask your partner to consciously feel his or her pain during the treatment to verify the success of your efforts.

Foot Reflexology

In the case of severe, acute back pain, it is sometimes impossible to carry out a foot reflexology massage, because the recipient may not be able to lie on his or her back. However, for chronic back pain, regular treatment—perhaps twice a week—can help.

The back is represented on both soles along the inside edges of the feet (the edges that face one another). These areas are easy to locate and easy to treat using the blunt end of the gem stick. Proceed with caution, because this can be painful for the recipient. Massage the appropriate areas on each foot for 5 minutes. Afterward, ask the recipient to get up and tell you whether or not the pain has subsided. Your partner should notice at least a small improvement after this treatment.

If you find an especially painful spot, carefully massage it using the pointed end of the stick. Remain on this point for 2 to 3 minutes. You may have found the exact vertebra responsible for the pain.

In the spirit of a holistic approach, it can also be helpful to massage the whole body on both soles of the feet, spending 5 minutes on each foot. Check your partner's perception of the pain again after this.

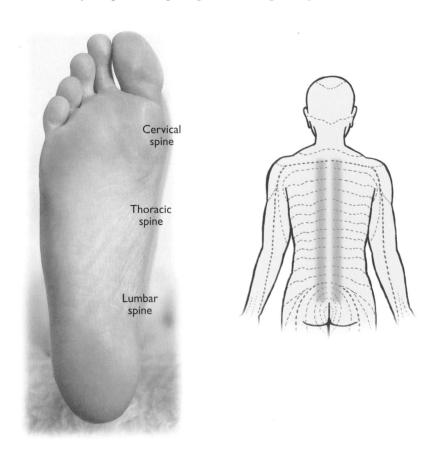

Accompanying Holistic Therapies

Acupressure is generally more helpful than any other measure. However, using muscle and joint massage oil and the blunt end of the gem stick, you can try massaging the muscles in the narrow area directly to the left and the right of the spine. The focus of the treatment should be in the painful part of the back. If lying down causes your partner too much pain, you can administer the massage with the recipient in a seated position.

Placing a warming pillow or a hot-water bottle on the back in the evening can also be soothing.

Coughs and Other Lung Ailments

Acupressure can help with a number of problems affecting the lungs. For serious illnesses, such as pneumonia, acupressure will usually not suffice as a single therapy. However, it can help alleviate pain and will contribute to the healing process. Acupressure can also help with symptoms of bronchial asthma and bronchitis, but for bronchitis, a plant-based expectorant (herbal remedy for coughs) is usually necessary to help expel phlegm.

If the problem is a cough caused by allergies, acupressure can help alleviate the symptoms. However, because the cause of the cough is the allergy, this is a difficult problem for amateurs to treat.

Preferred stones: Rock crystal cleanses the mucous membranes, reduces inflammation, and helps in general with infection. Fluorite also has beneficial effects on mucous membranes. Rutile quartz and aventurine help alleviate lung problems. Heliotrope strengthens the immune system.

Ear Acupressure

First locate and treat the two general points in the ear. One of these is located at the tip of the triangle in the upper part of the ear, the other on the center axis of the ear. Treating the antidepressant point, at the end of the ridge at the edge of the ear, is also soothing.

The points for the lungs and bronchi are in very close proximity to one another, making it a simple matter to treat a variety of respiratory ailments. The important points are located in the deeper area of the ear

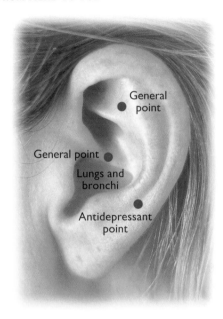

just above the earlobe. Search this area for painful points and treat all points you find for 10 to 20 seconds on each ear. Proceed with care, since this area is very sensitive to pain. Between applications, ask the recipient whether he or she can feel any improvement. Treat twice a day as needed.

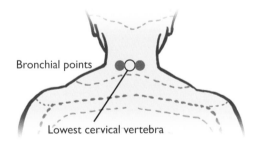

Body Acupressure

The two most important body acupressure points for the lungs and bronchi are easy to locate. With clothing removed from the torso, examine the cervical spine to find the vertebra that protrudes the most (the lowest cervical vertebra). To check that you have found it, touch it with a finger and have your partner turn his or her head; the vertebra will remain stationary.

Half a finger's width on each side of this vertebra, you will find the two spots to treat. Press the pointed end of the gem stick on each side for 2 to 3 minutes, one after the other. Make sure that you are not causing the recipient too much pain. Treat twice a day as needed.

Combine this body acupressure treatment with ear acupressure or foot reflexology. Reflexology massage may also be helpful.

Foot Reflexology

On the soles of the feet, the area corresponding to the bronchi and the lungs is rather large and easy to find. Massage the whole area with the blunt end of the gem stick for about 10 minutes on each foot. Move through the area in circles, spending extra time on painful spots. The massage should be perceived as pleasant. Ask your partner several times during the massage whether the pain is getting better.

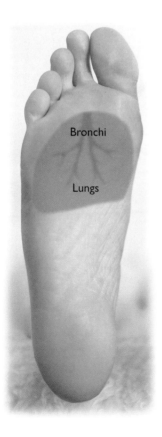

Reflexology Massage

A reflexology massage can be very soothing, especially since respiratory problems are often accompanied by tensions in the back, most of the time in the thoracic spine area. Accordingly, focus your efforts in this area.

Massage only the narrow area to the left and right of the thoracic spine for about 20 minutes, using the blunt end of the gem stick. If your partner also has pain in the lower back, you can continue the treatment farther down along the back.

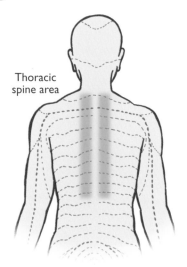

Thoracic
spine area

Accompanying Holistic Therapies

To help expel phlegm, an herbal expectorant (such as thyme tea or another herbal remedy good for coughs) will help. It is also important to drink plenty of liquids to loosen the phlegm, since thick phlegm is not easily expelled.

Rib and Chest Pain

Shingles, an inflammatory condition caused by a virus, is a common cause for pain in the rib area. This pain can be very severe. An acute itch and slight pain between the ribs may indicate the onset of an attack. In some cases, especially among older people, the healing process can take months or years. In the worst cases, the pain remains even after the skin eruptions have disappeared.

Regular acupressure treatment can help alleviate rib pain due to shingles and other causes, including bruised or broken ribs. These also can cause a great deal of pain, and heal more quickly when treated with acupressure.

Preferred stones: Amethyst and sodalite alleviate nerve pain. Rock crystal reduces inflammation and is effective in general against illness. Fluorite has beneficial effects against nerve-related pain, including shingles.

Ear Acupressure

First locate and treat the two general points in the ear. One of these is located at the tip of the triangle in the upper part of the ear, the other on the center axis of the ear. Treating the antidepressant point, located at the end of the ridge at the edge of the ear, will also be pleasant for the recipient.

In the ear, the rib area is located to the left and right of the edge on which the thoracic spine is reflected. Search this area and the edge itself for pain-sensitive points. Keep in mind that because the ribs enclose the lungs, you might find sensitive points in the lung area as well.

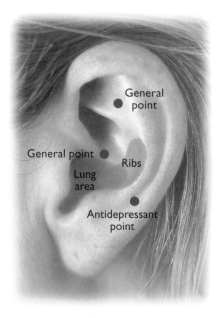

The ribs and the spaces between them can hurt even if the person is not moving. Often, breathing alone will be painful. To verify the success of your treatment, ask your partner to tell you if the pain is subsiding.

In the case of severe pain, perform this treatment twice a day for 10 to 15 minutes at a time.

Foot Reflexology

Since the ribs enclose the lungs, massage the lung area on the sole of each foot for about 10 to 15 minutes, using the blunt end of the gem stick. Spend extra time on painful spots.

If the pain is concentrated on one point, as the result of a fall, for example, you can carefully treat a particularly pain-sensitive spot with the pointed end of the gem stick. Spend 2 minutes on this point, but do not apply very much pressure, since the soles of the feet can be very sensitive. Between applications, ask your partner to tell you if the pain is subsiding.

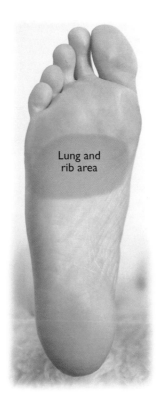

Lung and
rib area

Reflexology Massage

Do not perform reflexology massage for shingles. For other problems in this area, however, reflexology massage can help alleviate pain.

If you have ever seen a human skeleton (or a picture of a skeleton), you may have noticed that the ribs run on a slightly downward slant from back to front. You may be able to feel this on your own body; try running a finger along one of your ribs.

Thus, if there is a painful spot on the front of the ribs, the respective reflex zone is located slightly higher on the back. Accordingly, massage an area that is somewhat higher than that of the pain, to both the left and the right of the spine. Always massage both sides, even if the pain is limited to one side of the body.

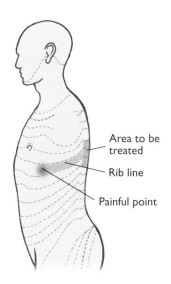

Area to be treated

Rib line

Painful point

Accompanying Holistic Therapies

Massaging the painful spot may not accomplish much. Instead, it may be helpful to simply place the gem stick lengthwise on the painful spot and leave it there for about 30 minutes.

Bruises and sprains should be iced several times a day for the first two days, after which warmth usually is better. Apply muscle and joint massage oil to the ribs several times a day. For acute injuries, take

3 pellets per hour of the homeopathic remedy Arnica D6 or D12.

In the case of shingles, it is important to see a doctor. Supplementing with vitamins B_1 and B_6 may help.

Heart Problems

There are many causes for pain in the area of the heart. Heart problems can be very serious, so it is important to consult a doctor about unexplained pain in the heart area, especially if it occurs frequently. Keep in mind that even severe heart problems sometimes cause only small amounts of pain.

If the pain occurs after eating, it may be caused by fullness of the stomach or large intestine. This can exert pressure on the heart and cause it to move slightly on its axis. A treatment of the stomach and intestinal area is necessary in such cases.

Heart disturbances, such as irregular and accelerated heartbeats, may be alleviated with acupressure. Sometimes such disturbances occur because of fear or excitement, but often, there is no obvious cause. Before undertaking acupressure, the recipient should see a doctor for diagnosis of any serious underlying heart condition.

Preferred stones: Rose quartz and aventurine are beneficial for the heart. Amethyst and aventurine help alleviate anxiety and pain. Rutile quartz gives strength and lessens fear. Sodalite has calming qualities.

Ear Acupressure

First locate and treat the two general points in the ear. One of these is located at the tip of the triangle in the upper part of the ear, the other on the center axis of the ear. Treating the antidepressant point, located at the end of the ridge at the edge of the ear, and the two relaxation points will also be pleasant for the recipient.

Because the heart is relatively small, the heart points are located close to one another in the middle of the deeper part of the ear. Proceed with caution, as this spot can be very sensitive to pain.

Treat both ears, not just the ear on the left side. The heart is located in the center of the body in the left part of the chest, so part of it is reflected in the right ear.

In the case of an acute heart disturbance, a single treatment may help. For chronic heart problems, perform the treatment two or three times a week. Ear acupressure can be combined to good effect with reflexology massage.

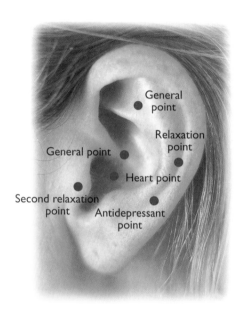

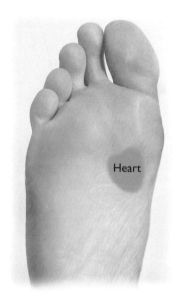

Foot Reflexology
In the spirit of a holistic approach, it can be helpful to treat the entire body on both soles of the feet. Look for points that are sensitive to pressure and treat them with the blunt end of the gem stick.

The focus of the treatment, however, is on massaging the heart area. Apply slightly stronger pressure here, since the intention is to calm the heart.

Reflexology Massage
Nerves that come from the spine innervate the heart as well as its large arteries and veins. Massage the entire thoracic spine area for 20 to

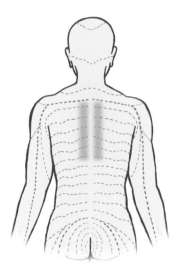

30 minutes, using the blunt end of the gem stick. If you want, use the calming lavender massage oil while doing this.

Accompanying Holistic Therapies

Valerian may be soothing for heart disturbances and accompanying anxiety.

Always remember the importance of proper diagnosis by a medical professional.

Low Blood Pressure and Other Circulation Problems

There is little one can do against low blood pressure, and acupressure will have an effect only after extended treatment. However, if you suspect circulatory collapse or any serious heart or circulation problem, do not hesitate to call for an ambulance.

On the sole of the foot, there is a particularly effective acupressure point that is helpful against circulatory collapse as well as low blood pressure. If you suspect circulatory collapse, perform acupressure on the sole of the foot as described on the following page, under Body Acupressure, and call for medical help immediately.

Preferred stones: Rose quartz benefits heart ailments of all kinds and helps promote good blood circulation. Rock crystal boosts energy. Heliotrope provides strength and supports good blood circulation, and rutile quartz gives stability. Amethyst and sodalite have calming effects.

Ear Acupressure

For low blood pressure, examine the entire ear for sensitive points and treat each one for about 10 seconds. When performed regularly, this holistic approach to ear acupressure can stabilize the entire body and its circulation.

Body Acupressure

There is a particularly effective acupressure point on the sole of the foot that can be used in the case of acute circulatory collapse as well as for low blood pressure. This point is part of body acupuncture, but must not be poked with a needle, since the pain would be unbearable. In Chinese emergency medicine, there are acupuncturists who can interrupt circulatory collapse by administering a sharp, focused slap to this point on the sole of the foot.

The point is relatively easy to find, because it lies in a small groove in the upper part of the sole of the foot. Press the blunt end of the gem stick against this spot for a few seconds. Only in absolute emergencies should you use the pointed end of the gem stick, but even then, proceed with great caution, because this will cause a lot of pain.

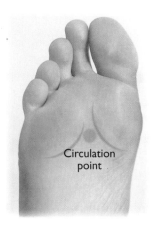

Circulation
point

Accompanying Holistic Therapies

The homeopathic remedy Camphor, taken as drops of tincture, can lead to a short-term increase in blood pressure.

Stomach Problems

Stomach pains, particularly in the upper stomach, are very common and may or may not be accompanied by nausea and vomiting. Such pain may be due to infection or simply excitement that has "upset" the stomach.

The large intestine, which passes close to the stomach, may cause discomfort in the upper stomach area. Occasionally, gallbladder problems can be confused with stomach problems. Since all of these organs are located very close to one another in the abdomen, successful acupressure treatment does not depend upon an accurate diagnosis. However, as with all health problems, it is best to seek professional medical attention to be sure that there is no serious underlying illness.

Preferred stones: Fluorite has beneficial effects on the mucous membranes. Amethyst calms and alleviates pain, and rock crystal fends off illness. Aventurine, amethyst, and rutile quartz help to relax the body during times of stress. Sodalite is helpful for digestive tract disorders.

Ear Acupressure

First locate and treat the two general points in the ear. One of these is located at the tip of the triangle in the upper part of the ear, the other on the center axis of the ear. Treating the antidepressant point, at the end of the ridge at the edge of the ear, will also be pleasant for the recipient.

In the deeper part of the ear, around the ridge, is the area that corresponds to the stomach. Search this area for sensitive points and treat them with the pointed end of the gem stick. Immediate results may be noticeable, so be sure to check with your partner to see if he or she feels improvement. If necessary, examine the adjacent intestinal area for sensitive spots and treat these as well.

When performed several times a day, ear acupressure can be very effective for acute stomach and intestinal upsets. For best results, treat chronic stomach ailments two or three times a week.

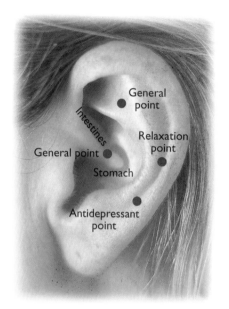 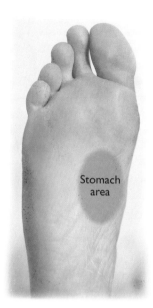

Foot Reflexology

In the spirit of holistic treatment, it can be helpful to treat the whole body on both soles of the feet, paying special attention to sensitive spots.

The area that corresponds to the stomach is located on the sole just below the ball of the foot. Massage this area, with the blunt end of the gem stick, on both feet for 5 minutes each. Ask your partner between massages whether he or she is feeling any better.

In the case of diarrhea or constipation, the direction of your massage is important. For more information, see Intestinal Cramps, Constipation, and Diarrhea starting on page 84.

Reflexology Massage

For chronic stomach ailments, regular reflexology massage can provide beneficial support to the affected area.

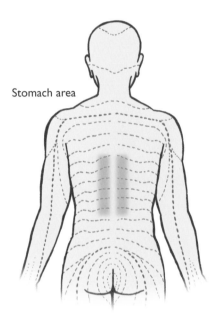

Stomach area

The nerves of the lower thoracic spine area also innervate the stomach. Apply massage oil and massage the thoracic spine area for about 20 minutes. In the case of a nervous, upset stomach, use lavender massage oil.

Accompanying Holistic Therapies

Chamomile and licorice tea help fight infections, although people with high blood pressure should not take licorice tea. Chamomile tea helps soothe stomach upsets of all kinds. Peppermint and ginger tea help against nausea.

Liver and Gallbladder Ailments

Liver and gallbladder problems are very common. They are often accompanied by feelings of fullness in the stomach area. Such problems are often linked to overeating, an unhealthy diet high in fat, or excessive consumption of alcohol, all of which can lead to a fatty liver. Gallstones may cause discomfort, but sometimes remain undetected. If they do not cause any discomfort, gallstones do not necessarily require treatment.

Regardless of the cause, acupressure can help alleviate the pain and discomfort, even in cases of severe, painful bilious colic.

Preferred stones: Amethyst alleviates pain. Fluorite has beneficial effects for the mucous membranes, and rock crystal fights illness in general.

Ear Acupressure

First locate and treat the two general points in the ear. One of these is located at the tip of the triangle in the upper part of the ear, the other on the center axis of the ear.

The gallbladder is located in the lower body part, near where the liver is reflected in the ear.

After a treatment using the sharp end of the gem stick on each point for 20 to 30 seconds, you should notice a rapid improvement in the patient's condition. Ask the recipient how he or she is feeling.

For acute gallbladder pain, ear acupressure can be very beneficial and should be administered several times a day. Treat chronic liver and gallbladder ailments two or three times a week.

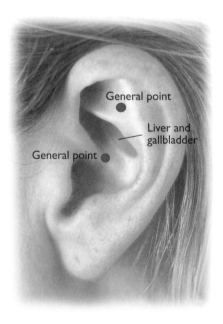

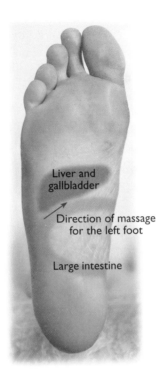

Liver and gallbladder

Direction of massage for the left foot

Large intestine

Foot Reflexology

The liver and gallbladder are located almost in the middle of the sole of the foot. Massage this area on both feet for 5 minutes each with the blunt end of the gem stick. In cases of acute pain, ask your partner during the treatment whether he or she is feeling better.

Gallbladder problems are sometimes connected with constipation. If this is the case, massage the area of the large intestine, making sure that you massage in the natural direction of the intestine, from top to bottom on the right sole and bottom to top on the left sole. Otherwise, you may worsen the constipation. For more information, see Intestinal Cramps, Constipation, and Diarrhea starting on page 84.

Treat chronic liver and gallbladder problems two or three times a week. In the spirit of holistic therapy, it can be helpful to treat the entire body on both soles of the feet. Look for spots that are sensitive to pressure.

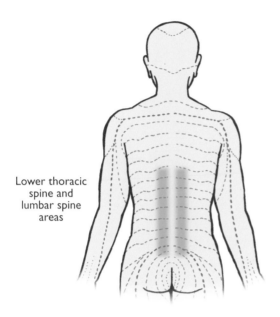

Lower thoracic
spine and
lumbar spine
areas

Reflexology Massage

Perform reflexology massage after ear acupressure or foot reflexology. With chronic ailments, regular massage with the gem stick can bring about lasting improvement. Because liver and gallbladder ailments are often accompanied by digestive problems, the stomach and intestinal areas should be included in the treatment.

Massage the area to the left and right of the lower thoracic spine area and the entire lumbar spine area for about 20 minutes.

Accompanying Holistic Therapies

Peppermint, cumin, and dandelion root teas all stimulate the gallbladder, which can help reduce feelings of fullness after a high-fat meal. Cumin and fennel tea can also help with flatulence.

If gallbladder problems originate with the liver, extract of milk thistle seed (*Silybum marianum*) can be helpful if taken over an extended period of time. Follow the manufacturer's directions for dosage.

Intestinal Cramps, Constipation, and Diarrhea

The upper area of the small intestine does not contain pain-transmitting nerves, so pain in the stomach area is often related to the large intestine. Since the main function of the large intestine is to thicken the stool, this is where diarrhea and constipation problems usually originate.

Gallbladder problems may also result in painful flatulence. Thus, when treating problems in the intestines, it may also be necessary to treat the liver and gallbladder.

Preferred stones: Aventurine and amethyst are calming, helping to relieve cramps and alleviate pain. Rock crystal is good against illness in general and, because it helps with paralysis, acts against the intestinal sluggishness that can contributes to constipation. Fluorite has beneficial effects on mucous membranes.

Ear Acupressure

First locate and treat the two general points in the ear. One of these is located at the tip of the triangle in the upper part of the ear, the other on the center axis of the ear.

Unfortunately, because the part of the ear that corresponds to the intestines is located under the edge of the ear close to the temples, it can be difficult to treat the entire intestinal area with the pointed end of a gem stick. If necessary, you can use a paper clip bent into an open position to gently treat this hidden part. (This is better than administering no treatment at all.) Treatment should bring about a rapid, observable improvement. Check with your partner to find out if his or her symptoms have improved.

Applied several times a day, ear acupressure can be especially effective for acute intestinal problems. Treat chronic intestinal ailments two or three times a week.

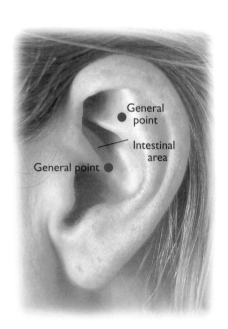

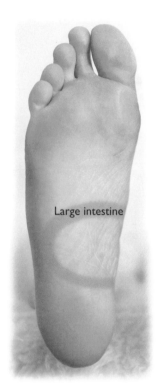

Foot Reflexology

Regular foot reflexology can be helpful in alleviating chronic intestinal ailments, including diarrhea. The area corresponding to the large intestine can be easily found on the sole of the foot and is well placed for treatment. It is located around the arch of the foot, creating an arc from below the ball of the foot to the top of the heel.

For constipation, applying gentle pressure with the blunt end of the gem stick, massage this area on the left sole from bottom to top and on the right sole from top to bottom. The reverse is true for diarrhea: Using stronger pressure, massage the left sole from the top of the area to the bottom and the right sole from bottom to top. The exception is acute diarrhea, in which the pathogen must exit the intestine. In such a case, massage in the direction indicated for constipation, but do so less intensively.

The massage for either constipation or diarrhea should last about 10 minutes. In the spirit of a holistic approach, it can be helpful to treat the entire body on both soles of the foot, paying special attention to pain-sensitive areas.

Reflexology Massage

Chronic intestinal ailments can be influenced via the nerves on the back when you use reflexology massage in combination with ear acupressure or foot reflexology massage. For best results, administer reflexology massage once or twice a week as needed.

Massage the area to the left and right of the lower thoracic spine and the entire lumbar spine area for about 20 minutes with the blunt end of the gem stick.

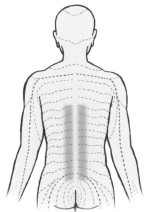

Accompanying Holistic Therapies

For acute diarrhea, take dissolved charcoal tablets or a probiotic supplement (for example, acidophilus) to help eliminate the pathogen that is causing the illness.

For constipation, be sure that the diet contains an adequate amount of fiber. Drinking enough water is also essential. Laxatives are not a good solution, because over time they suppress the intestines' ability to function properly and may one day stop working.

Menstrual Problems

Menstrual cramps are a common problem among women of childbearing age. Each month, the uterus expels the mucous membrane lining that has built up during the previous month, which leads to menstrual bleeding. This mucous membrane lining is naturally renewed every month and plays an important role in pregnancy. Many girls and women know little about the actual process and curse the discomfort caused by this miracle of nature.

Menstrual cramps can be quite severe, and pain-relieving drugs often do not suffice to ease the pain. Some doctors even prescribe oral contraceptive pills, which decrease the menstrual flow and associated pain. However, before resorting to this step, a woman who suffers severe cramps might want to consider acupressure and reflexology, which can be very effective in relieving symptoms.

Preferred stones: Rose quartz is especially effective for women's problems. Fluorite benefits the mucous membranes, and amethyst alleviates pain. Heliotrope relaxes uterine cramping and encourages the production of new blood to balance the blood loss of menstruation.

Ear Acupressure

Administered several times a day, ear acupressure can be especially effective for acute menstrual cramp pain.

First locate and treat the two general points in the ear. One is located at the tip of the triangle in the upper part of the ear, the other on the

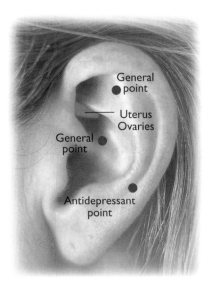

center axis of the ear. In addition, treating the antidepressant point at the end of the ridge on the edge of the ear is always appreciated.

Depending on the shape of the recipient's ear, it can be difficult to reach the correct spot with the pointed end of the gem stick, because the point is located under the edge of the ear close to the temples. If necessary, you can use a paper clip bent into an open position to gently treat this hidden part.

After treatment, you should observe a rapid improvement in symptoms. To guide your treatment, ask the recipient to tell you about changes in the intensity of the pain as you work.

Foot Reflexology

The reproductive organs are located on the sole of the foot on the inside edge of the heel. Look for sensitive areas and massage these using the blunt edge of the gem stick.

In the spirit of a holistic approach, it can be very helpful to treat the whole body on both soles of the feet.

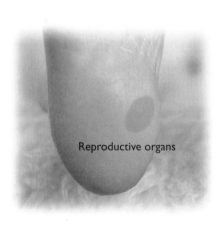
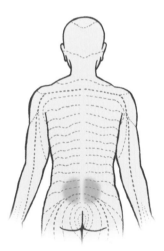

Reproductive organs

Reflexology Massage

Use muscle and joint massage oil and the blunt end of the gem stick for this massage. Massage the lumbar spine over a broad area for about 10 minutes. Often, menstrual discomfort is associated with pain in this area of the back, and this treatment will address this pain as well.

Combine reflexology massage with foot reflexology once or twice a week for a holistic treatment for chronic menstrual problems.

Accompanying Holistic Therapies

When taken regularly over several months, the herbal remedy chasteberry (*Vitex agnus-castus*) usually helps relieve menstrual problems.

Bladder and Kidney Problems

In very hot weather, an adult can produce more than 5 quarts of sweat a day. To replace this quantity of lost fluid, one may have to consume as much as 7 quarts of water. This is an extreme example, but in my daily work I notice time and again that most people do not drink enough water. According to one rule of thumb, a person who weighs 155 pounds should drink about 5 pints of liquid a day, preferably water. (Milk, soft drinks, coffee, and black, oolong, or green tea do not count toward this daily amount.)

In people who do not drink enough water, bacteria can easily reproduce in the bladder. This may lead to an infection of the bladder, which in turn can ascend to the renal pelvis and kidneys, causing a more serious problem.

Of course, there are many other causes for bladder and renal pelvis infections. Because the bladder and kidneys work in concert but are located in different parts of the body, you must treat both areas. The kidneys and bladder are connected by the two ureters (tubes that carry urine from the kidneys to the bladder), which can also cause problems.

In the case of infection, acupressure alleviates pain immediately, but only rarely suffices as a stand-alone therapy.

Preferred stones: Fluorite has good effects on the mucous membranes. Rock crystal is effective in general against infections and illness and reduces mucous membrane inflammation. Rose quartz and heliotrope support good blood circulation. Amethyst alleviates pain.

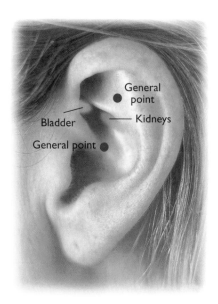

Ear Acupressure

First locate and treat the two general points in the ear. One of these is located at the tip of the triangle in the upper part of the ear, the other on the center axis of the ear.

Always treat both the kidney and bladder areas, as well as the area between them that corresponds to the ureter, even if only the bladder is affected.

It can be difficult to reach the correct spot with the pointed end of the gem stick, because the point is located under the edge of the ear close to the temples. If necessary, you can use a paper clip bent into an open position to gently treat this hidden part. (This is better than no treatment at all.) Treat each point for 20 to 30 seconds. After treatment, you should see a rapid improvement. Ask your partner to verify this.

For an acute bladder, renal pelvis, or kidney infection, apply ear acupressure several times a day. Treat chronic bladder and kidney problems two or three times a week.

Foot Reflexology

Treat chronic bladder and kidney problems two or three times a week. In the spirit of a holistic approach, it can be helpful to treat the whole

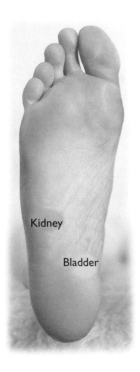

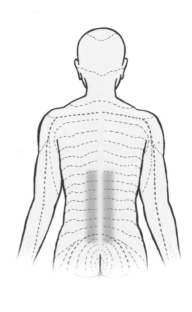

body on both soles of the feet. Be alert for pain-sensitive spots.

The kidney and bladder are located in different areas of the feet. Remember also to treat the part between these two points, which corresponds to the ureter. Search for pain-sensitive spots in the entire lower body area and massage with the blunt end of the gem stick for 5 to 10 minutes.

Reflexology Massage

Combine a reflexology massage of the entire lumbar and lower thoracic spine areas with ear acupressure or foot reflexology.

The kidneys are not always where they should be, although this only rarely causes problems. You may simply have to include the middle of the thoracic spine area in your gem stick massage.

Accompanying Holistic Therapies

The most important additional therapy is to drink plenty of liquids. This may include an herbal tea formulated specifically for bladder or kidney problems, a nettle leaf (*Urtica dioica*) tea, or cranberry juice.

If urination causes a burning sensation, it can be helpful to take 3 pellets of the homeopathic preparation Cantharis D6 or D12 once an hour.

Hip Problems

Many older people suffer from hip pain, which can be quite severe. In many cases, arthrosis destroys the cartilage of the joint. Artificial hips can be inserted relatively easily, but some do not last very long, and these procedures are often delayed. Fracture of the femoral neck (the top part of the thighbone) is also common in older people. This bone is located very close to the hip joint.

Ear acupressure can help ease the pain of these and all other hip problems.

Preferred stones: Amethyst alleviates pain. Rose quartz and heliotrope support good blood circulation, and rock crystal is effective in general against illnesses. Rutile quartz releases tensions and provides the stability one needs to "stand on one's own two feet." Fluorite helps with pain related to arthritis and arthrosis.

Ear Acupressure

First locate and treat the two general points in the ear. One of these is located at the tip of the triangle in the upper part of the ear, the other on the center axis of the ear.

Unfortunately, the hip is somewhat difficult to find on the ear. You will have to examine a rather large area for pain-sensitive spots. During treatment, take a break and ask your partner to get up and walk around to verify that you have found the right point. If you note an improvement, continue treating the points you located and treated immediately previously.

Sometimes, especially with acute hip pain, hip and back problems are difficult to distinguish from one another. Thus, you should also locate and treat the area of the lumbar spine. Here, too, you should check in with your partner to guide the success of your treatment. If your partner notices improvement only after you treat the lumbar spine area,

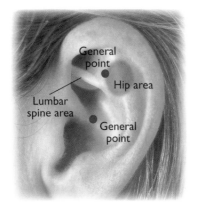
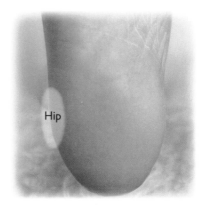

you may conclude that the affected area is the back, with pain radiating to the hips.

Foot Reflexology

In keeping with a holistic approach, it can help to regularly treat the whole body on both soles of the feet, especially if arthrosis is the cause of the hip pain. Be alert for pain-sensitive points.

The hips themselves are located on the outside of the heels. Massage these small areas with the blunt end of the gem stick, using circular movements.

Reflexology Massage

Massage, with the blunt end of the gem stick, the lower lumbar vertebra area and a part of the lower-lying sacral area. As part of holistic

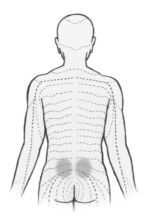

treatment, also massage the areas to the left and right of the entire spine on a regular basis.

Accompanying Holistic Therapies

Drinking 3 cups a day of nettle leaf tea (*Urtica dioica*) helps to reduce the buildup of toxins. In the long run, a devil's claw (*Harpagophytum procumbens*) preparation can help alleviate pain.

Thigh Pain

Pain in the thigh can be related to back pain. The sciatic nerve runs along the thigh and is a common cause of pain down the back of the thigh. Sport injuries and vein infections can also cause problems in the thighs. Regardless of the cause, however, acupressure can help ease pain.

Preferred stones: Amethyst alleviates pain and relieves tension. Heliotrope and rose quartz encourage good blood circulation. Rock crystal is helpful against inflammation and paralysis.

Ear Acupressure

First locate and treat the two general points in the ear. One of these is located at the tip of the triangle in the upper part of the ear, the other on the center axis of the ear.

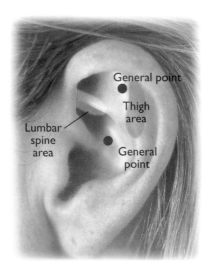

The area that corresponds to the thigh is large, and the points are difficult to locate. Ask your partner to get up and walk around between treatment applications so you can determine whether you have found the right points. If you notice improvement, resume treating the points on which you were working immediately previously.

If the cause of the pain is the sciatic nerve, locate and treat the lumbar spine area. Here, too, you will have to check in with your partner during treatment to verify the success of the therapy.

For acute pain, perform the treatment twice a day. For chronic pain, treat two or three times a week.

Foot Reflexology

When the cause of thigh pain originates in the back, it helps to massage the relevant area of the foot. The lumbar spine area is located on the inside edge of the sole, near the heel. Look for pain-sensitive spots in this area and massage them, using the blunt end of the gem stick.

If you find an especially painful spot, carefully massage it using the pointed end of the stick. Remain on this point for 2 to 3 minutes. You may have found the exact vertebra responsible for the pain.

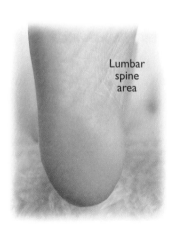

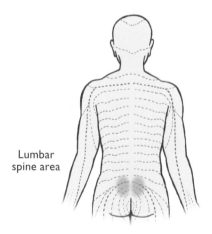

Reflexology Massage

Using muscle massage oil, perform reflexology massage with the gem stick after ear acupressure or foot reflexology. Massage the lumbar spine area, because some of the nerves that originate here run along the thigh and can cause pain there.

Accompanying Holistic Therapies

Since the potential causes of thigh pain are so varied, it is difficult to pinpoint helpful accompanying therapies. If the problem is localized (for example, due to a muscle tear), you can massage the affected area locally with the blunt end of the gem stick. Be careful, because this massage should be perceived as pleasant. In some cases, it may be better to simply place the gem stick lengthwise on the affected area and allow it to rest there for 20 to 30 minutes.

Rubbing the affected area with muscle and joint massage oil can also be soothing.

For acute injuries, it can be helpful to take 3 pellets per hour of the homeopathic preparation Arnica D12. Apply ice to acute injuries and vein infections.

Knee Problems

The knee is a complicated joint under severe stress. Because of this constant stress, many people have pain and other problems with their knees. The causes of knee pain are extremely varied, and corrective surgery may be required in some cases.

Regardless of the cause or severity, however, ear acupressure can help alleviate knee pain. For minor knee problems, acupressure alone may be sufficient to provide relief.

Preferred stones: Amethyst alleviates pain and relieves tension. Rock crystal reduces inflammation. Rose quartz and heliotrope support good blood circulation.

Ear Acupressure

First locate and treat the two general points in the ear. One is located at the tip of the triangle in the upper part of the ear, the other on the center axis of the ear.

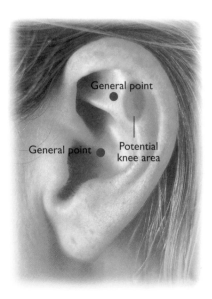

The area in the ear that represents the knee is relatively large and the correct points will be located in a slightly different place for each person. Search this entire area and treat all pain-sensitive points that you find. Have your partner move his or her knee—he or she may want to get up and walk around—between treatment applications so you can determine whether you have found the right spots. A patient, thorough massage of this area with the tip of the gem stick can be very effective in alleviating acute knee pain.

Accompanying Holistic Therapies

If you choose to massage the painful area of the knee itself, proceed with great caution, using the blunt end of the gem stick. Do not treat protruding bones. Rub the knee with muscle and joint massage oil several times a day.

Ice acute knee injuries several times a day during the first two days. After that, application of warmth is better. The homeopathic preparation Arnica D12, taken at a dosage of 3 pellets per hour, can be helpful for acute injuries.

Lower Leg Pain

Injuries to the shin are extremely painful and can be alleviated with ear acupressure. Acupressure can also help support the healing of broken bones and relieve pain related to varicose veins and vein infections.

Frequently recurring calf cramps are usually caused by a lack of magnesium, and must be treated accordingly to effect any long-term change.

Preferred stones: Aventurine and amethyst alleviate pain and relieve tension. Rock crystal is effective against inflammation. Rose quartz and heliotrope support good blood circulation.

Ear Acupressure

Lower leg problems are rarely chronic. As such, you need only locate and treat the points in the ear that correspond to the lower leg. Unfortunately, as with all extremities of the body, the lower leg area can be difficult to find, as the correct points will be located in a slightly different place for each person.

Search for and treat painful points in the upper inner part of the ear with the tip of the gem stick. Periodically ask your partner to tell you

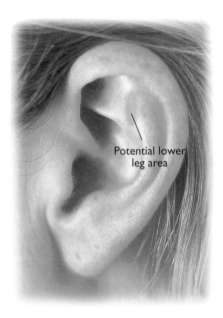

Potential lower leg area

whether or not the pain is subsiding. He or she will probably not need to move the leg in order to notice the improvement.

Accompanying Holistic Therapies

Rub the affected area several times a day with muscle and joint massage oil. You can massage the calf using the blunt end of the gem stick and muscle massage oil, but not the shin. Local massage of the painful area must be perceived as pleasant.

Ice acute injuries several times a day for the first two days. After that, application of warmth is usually better. The homeopathic preparation Arnica D12, taken at a dosage of 3 pellets per hour, can be helpful for acute injuries. Vein infections must be iced.

Supplementing with magnesium can be effective against recurring calf cramps. Calcium may sometimes help as well, but the two minerals should not be taken at the same time.

Ankle Problems

The ankle is vulnerable to torn tendons, sprains, tears, and breaks, and some of these injuries must be treated surgically. Unfortunately, most ankle injuries are long-term problems and require several treatments. Regardless of the cause, however, you can alleviate pain and support the healing process with ear acupressure.

Preferred stones: Amethyst alleviates pain. Rock crystal reduces inflammation. Heliotrope and rose quartz stimulate good blood circulation.

Ear Acupressure

First locate and treat the two general points in the ear. One is located at the tip of the triangle in the upper part of the ear, the other on the center axis of the ear.

The ankle joint is fairly easy to find in the tip of the ear. Locate sensitive points and ask your partner to move his or her foot during treatment. If the pain in the ankle subsides during treatment, remain on that point until no further improvement occurs. Because your partner can

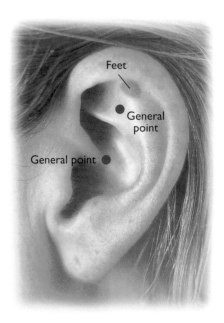

move his or her foot *while* you are treating a particular point, it is easier to gauge what is working best to alleviate the pain.

For acute pain, treat several times a day. Perform regular treatment (two or three times a week) for chronic joint problems.

Accompanying Holistic Therapies

Ice injuries, such as sprains and torn tendons, several times a day for the first two days. After this time, application of warmth is usually better. Rub the joint with muscle and joint massage oil several times a day.

For acute injuries, the homeopathic preparation Arnica D12, taken at a dosage of 3 pellets per hour, can be helpful.

Foot and Toe Pain

Arthrosis in the base joint of the big toe can cause severe pain, especially among older people. A bunion or so-called hammertoe, in which the big toe becomes severely bent, can also be very painful. Equally uncomfortable are deformed toes, which can develop even if one wears healthy shoes throughout one's life.

In order for ear acupressure to be successful, however, determining the cause of foot and toe pain is not important. Acupressure will support healing of acute problems and help relieve any pain.

Preferred stones: Amethyst alleviates pain, and rock crystal reduces inflammation. Heliotrope and rose quartz encourage good blood circulation. Fluorite helps with pain related to arthritis and arthrosis.

Ear Acupressure

First locate and treat the two general points in the ear. One is located at the tip of the triangle in the upper part of the ear, the other on the center axis of the ear.

The toes are located at the very top of the ear and extend under the ear's outer edge. Since the edge is easy to move, it should not be difficult to reach this spot with the tip of your gem stick.

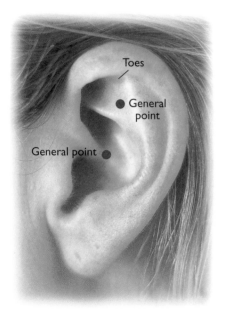

Foot Reflexology

In the spirit of a holistic approach, it can be helpful to regularly treat the whole body on the soles of both feet, especially for arthrosis. Be alert for pain-sensitive points, and treat them using the blunt end of the gem stick for 2 to 3 minutes each.

Accompanying Holistic Therapies

Drinking 3 cups a day of nettle leaf tea (*Urtica dioica*) can help the body eliminate toxins. In the long run, taking a devil's claw (*Harpagophytum procumbens*) preparation can also be effective against joint pain. Rub the toes several times a day with muscle and joint massage oil.

Ice acute injuries several times a day for the first two days, after which application of warmth is usually better. For acute injuries, the homeopathic remedy Arnica D12, taken at a dosage of 3 pellets per hour, can also be helpful.

Walking barefoot is healthy in general for the feet—unless, of course, one hits the leg of a table and breaks a toe in the process.

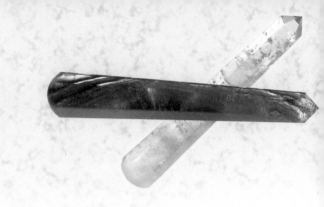

RESOURCES

Gem Sticks

Those who want to acquire the gem sticks used in this book may contact:

Heaven and Earth, LLC
P.O. Box 249
East Montpelier, VT 05651
802-476-4775
800-942-9423
heavenandearth@earthlink.net
www.heavenandearthjewelry.com

Books

Gienger, Michael. *Crystal Power, Crystal Healing*. London: Cassell & Co., 1998.

Hall, Judy. *The Crystal Bible*. Cincinnati: Walking Stick Press, 2004.

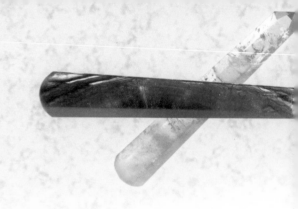

INDEX

Books of Related Interest

Facial Reflexology
A Self-Care Manual
by Marie-France Muller, M.D., N.D., Ph.D.

The Reflexology Atlas
by Bernard C. Kolster, M.D. and Astrid Waskowiak, M.D.

The Reflexology Manual
*An Easy-to-Use Illustrated Guide to the
Healing Zones of the Hands and Feet*
by Pauline Wills

The Healing Power of Gemstones
In Tantra, Ayurveda, and Astrology
by Harish Johari

The Mystery of the Crystal Skulls
Unlocking the Secrets of the Past, Present, and Future
by Chris Morton and Ceri Louise Thomas

The Stones of Time
Calendars, Sundials, and Stone Chambers of Ancient Ireland
by Martin Brennan

Pendulum Power
A Mystery You Can See, A Power You Can Feel
by Greg Nielsen and Joseph Polansky

The Aura-Soma Sourcebook
Color Therapy for the Soul
by Mike Booth with Carol McKnight

Inner Traditions • Bear & Company
P.O. Box 388
Rochester, VT 05767
1-800-246-8648
www.InnerTraditions.com

Or contact your local bookseller